A Feminist Ethnography of Secure Wards for Women with Learning Disabilities

T0384733

What is life like for women with learning disabilities detained in a secure unit? This book presents a unique ethnographic study conducted in a contemporary institution in England.

Rebecca Fish takes an interdisciplinary approach, drawing on both the social model of disability and intersectional feminist methodology, to explore the reasons why the women were placed in the unit, as well their experiences of day-to-day life as played out through relationships with staff and other residents. She raises important questions about the purpose of such units and the services they offer.

Through making the women's voices heard, this book presents their experiences and unique perspectives on topics such as seclusion, restraint, and resistance. Exploring how the ever present power disparity works to regulate women's behaviour, the book shows how institutional responses replicate women's bad experiences from the past, and how women's responses are seen as pathological. It demonstrates that women are not passive recipients of care, but shape their own identity and futures, sometimes by resisting the norms expected of them (within allowed limits) and sometimes by transgressing the rules. These insights thus challenge traditional institutional accounts of gender, learning disability and deviance and highlight areas for reform in policy, practice, methodology, and social theory.

This unique book will be of interest to scholars, students, policymakers and advocates working in the fields of learning disability and disability studies more widely, gender studies, and sociology.

Rebecca Fish has been working with people with learning disabilities since 1997. Her early work explored the meaning of self-harm for people with learning disabilities and the staff who work with them. Her work has informed policy and practice in the UK. She completed her PhD in 2015 and works as a researcher for the Centre for Disability Research at Lancaster University.

Interdisciplinary Disability Studies
Series editor: Mark Sherry, The University of Toledo, USA

For a full list of titles in this series, please visit www.routledge.com/series/ASH SER1401

Disability studies has made great strides in exploring power and the body. This series extends the interdisciplinary dialogue between disability studies and other fields by asking how disability studies can influence a particular field. It will show how a deep engagement with disability studies changes our understanding of the following fields: sociology, literary studies, gender studies, bioethics, social work, law, education, or history. This ground-breaking series identifies both the practical and theoretical implications of such an interdisciplinary dialogue and challenges people in disability studies as well as other disciplinary fields to critically reflect on their professional praxis in terms of theory, practice, and methods.

Disability, Society and Assistive Technology
Bodil Ravneberg and Sylvia Söderström

Disability and Rurality
Identity, Gender and Belonging
Karen Soldatic and Kelley Johnson

Pedagogy, Disability and Communication
Applying Disability Studies in the Classroom
Edited by Michael Jeffress

A Feminist Ethnography of Secure Wards for Women with Learning Disabilities
Locked Away
Rebecca Fish

Forthcoming:

A Sociological Approach to Acquired Brain Injury and Identity
Jonathan Harvey

Disability and Postsocialism
Teodor Mladenov

A Feminist Ethnography of Secure Wards for Women with Learning Disabilities

Locked Away

Rebecca Fish

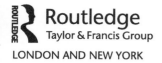
Routledge
Taylor & Francis Group

LONDON AND NEW YORK

First published 2018 by Routledge

2 Park Square, Milton Park, Abingdon, Oxfordshire OX14 4RN
52 Vanderbilt Avenue, New York, NY 10017

Routledge is an imprint of the Taylor & Francis Group, an informa business

First issued in paperback 2019

British Library Cataloguing-in-Publication Data
A catalogue record for this book is available from the British Library

Library of Congress Cataloging-in-Publication Data
Names: Fish, Rebecca, 1972– author.
Title: A feminist ethnography of secure wards for women with learning
    disabilities : locked away / Rebecca Fish.
Description: 1st Edition. | New York : Routledge, 2018. | Series:
    Interdisciplinary disability studies | Includes bibliographical references
    and index.
Identifiers: LCCN 2017037172 | ISBN 9781138088269 (hardback) |
    ISBN 9781315109985 (ebook)
Subjects: LCSH: Learning disabled women—Institutional care—
    Great Britain.
Classification: LCC HV3009.5.W65 F57 2018 | DDC
    362.3/850820941—dc23
LC record available at https://lccn.loc.gov/2017037172

ISBN: 978-1-138-08826-9 (hbk)
ISBN: 978-0-367-33894-7 (pbk)

Typeset in Times New Roman
by Apex CoVantage, LLC

Contents

Acknowledgements

I would like to say thank you to the women who lived at Unit C and the staff who worked with them. They were welcoming and open, generously sharing their stories and thoughts with me. Without them this book would not have been possible.

I would also like to thank the ESRC for funding this work, and Fiona Summers for encouraging me to apply for funding. Thank you to my colleagues and friends in the Centre for Gender and Women's Studies and the Centre for Disability Research at Lancaster University, for taking me on such an amazing journey.

I had the good fortune of being guided by the best supervisors imaginable for this study. Thank you Celia Roberts and Carol Thomas for such tremendous advice, guidance and insight.

I also had the pleasure of working with Hannah Morgan, as an extremely supportive colleague and friend, and Disability Studies Guru.

Thank you Adi, for giving me confidence to do this, for the inspiring daily discussions, and for taking on so many extra duties to free up my time. I am *indebted* and *grateful* to you in particular for manning the 'Thesaurus Helpline' service.

Thanks go to my boys: Sam, Thomas, Bruce, Isaac, Felix for the never-ending love and joy and for putting up with freezer-to-oven food on a regular basis. To Mum for all your love and faith, but also for the childcare, practical help and time you have given to me. To Emma for doing so much of our laundry, for the in-car ponderings, and for telling me often how proud of me you are. To Charlotte for the childcare, but more importantly for your kindness. To Sue for the encouraging messages, visits, thoughtful presents and silly cards.

The following people have given me invaluable help and encouragement: Mark Sherry, Susie Balderston, John Lobley, Liz Stitt, Helen Duperouzel, Brigit McWade, Cath Morton, Paula Johnson, Michaela Thomson, Maggie Mort, Debbie Phillips, Maureen McNeil, Rachael Lofthouse.

This book is dedicated to my mum, Stella and her sister Mary, for showing me what strong women are capable of.

Funding information

This study was completed with the financial support of an ESRC Nomination (Quota) Award Studentship (2010–2014) – ESRC Ref: ES/H037594/1

Existing publications from this study

Fish, R. (2013). Women who use secure services: Applying the literature to women with learning disabilities. *The Journal of Forensic Practice*, 15(3), 192–205. DOI: https://doi.org/10.1108/JFP-09-2012-0016

Fish, R. (2016). "They've said I'm vulnerable with men": Doing sexuality on locked wards. *Sexualities*, 19(5–6), 641–658. DOI: https://doi.org/10.1177/1363460715620574

Fish, R. (2016). Friends and Family: Relationships on the locked ward. *Disability and Society*, 31(10), 1385–1402. DOI: http://dx.doi.org/10.1080/09687599.2016.1261693

Fish, R. (2017). Researching experiences of learning disabled women on locked wards using ethnography. *Sage Research Methods Cases Part 2*. DOI: http://dx.doi.org/10.4135/9781526404411 Available at http://methods.sagepub.com/case/research ing-experiences-learning-disabled-women-locked-wards-ethnography (Accessed 09/12/2017).

Fish, R., and Hatton, C. (2017). Gendered experiences of physical restraint on locked wards for women. *Disability and Society*, 32(6), 790–809. DOI: http://dx.doi.org/10.10 80/09687599.2017.1329711

1   One year, one unit

This book is an ethnography of locked wards for women with learning disabilities. It represents just a small part of my life, the year of my fieldwork, when I spent time with people who live and work on the wards. However, for the women detained, this had been their day-to-day reality for years. These women had been removed, sometimes a great distance, from their families and friends, and compelled to lead a restricted life under surveillance and control.

The removal of people with learning disabilities from society has happened for generations in Western Europe and North America (Mansell and Ericsson, 1996). Despite the closure of large institutions in the 1980s and 1990s, and the 'resettling' of people into the community, the 2015 Learning Disability Census (HSCIC, 2015) found that there were around 3,000 people with learning disabilities in inpatient units or hospitals in England. My ethnography took place in one unit, but there are many relatively large units throughout the UK and new private ones are being built all the time (Brown et al., 2017). High profile coverage such as the Winterbourne View documentary (Chapman, 2011) and the Justice for LB inquiry (Ryan, 2017) shows that people can be subjected to abuse and neglect in these types of units, despite the large amount of money these placements cost.

Women with learning disabilities have been hidden away throughout history and characterised as 'failed women'. Although they are no longer institutionalised merely for being learning disabled, a crucial question is how much of this legacy remains? While reading the existing academic literature prior to my study, I noticed these women being portrayed as sheltered by families or staff, living with very traditional views about their abilities and the choices they can make in life. Imposed expectations become internalised by many women who accept the limitations, becoming passive and compliant. In my experience, these accounts do not represent women in locked units.

My study took place at an NHS secure unit for people with learning disabilities in the North of England; I have worked as a researcher in similar units for most of my career. My main interest prior to this ethnography had been exploring self-harm from the perspective of learning disabled women and the professionals who work with them (Duperouzel and Fish, 2010). Whilst doing this work, I became aware that the mainstream account was not a comprehensive portrayal – it simply did not represent the women that I had encountered. These were women who had been purposefully excluded from society because their behaviour deviates from normative expectations. I had often wondered how these women had ended up in a secure unit. What were their stories? How did they live out their lives, locked away from society? These questions were the inspiration for this book.

The purpose of this book, therefore, is to explore the experiences of learning disabled women detained in a British secure learning disability unit (I will call it Unit C for anonymity), and the staff who work with them. I use my own words and those of others gained from ethnographic research at three of the women's wards on the unit, in the form of fieldnotes and in-depth interview transcripts with both staff and clients.

I explore how women felt when first arriving at the unit, their relationships and daily life whilst living on the unit, their conceptions of progression and ideas about their future. I also look at the stories used by the staff to talk about the women who live on the unit, and the staff's perception of their own roles in relation to the women.

The social construction of labels

Although I write about my participants as 'having' learning disabilities or as 'learning disabled', I acknowledge these to be complex and controversial descriptions that are socially constructed. The category 'learning disabled' is defined on Unit C by IQ levels (below 70). In this respect, the label is arbitrarily designated by professionals (Rapley, 2004). The World Health Organization's categories of learning disability include IQ levels along with taxonomies of social functioning, and requirements for diagnosis to be within the developmental period (see O'Brien, 2001). Simpson's (1999) overview of the history of learning disability labels provides a critique of the classification mechanisms in use at particular times, as moving between physiological descriptions to social manifestations. He describes the association between changes in discourse and how society responds to learning disabled people, constituting them as objects of knowledge. Simpson describes the terminology as tactical and strategic, advancing institutional practices, and concludes that current service provision uses the concepts of behavioural (in)competence and (in)dependence to be central issues in defining people's needs.

The social construction of learning disability has been emphasised and critiqued by many scholars, and Rapley's (2004) work is particularly influential in this regard. Rapley stressed the power asymmetries which underlie the diagnostic process and the wider attribution of labels of incompetence and Otherness to learning disabled people. He regarded the power differentials between professionals and learning disabled people as 'the professional disenfranchisement' of learning disabled people (2004:5). Further, Jenkins (1998) brings to light the social construction of learning disability, noting that it is context-dependent and can be both accepted and contested in social interactions. Gill (2015:X) agrees with this, describing the diagnostic category as 'often nebulous and imprecise'. Although I acknowledge these terms to be contested (Gernsbacher, 2017), I use the terms 'learning disabilities' and 'learning disabled' because they are the dominant and accepted terminology in services such as the research site, and they locate my writing within the field of disability studies.

With reference to my use of the term 'client', I take into account the debate regarding terms for people who 'use' services (McLaughlin, 2009), notably the pervasiveness of business terminology into healthcare. McLaughlin finds most available terms problematic, due to the suggestion of 'choice' and marketisation within them, and calls for a new semantic system. Despite McLaughlin's claim that 'client' signifies the recipient position within a system of hierarchy, and even though it is clear that clients in Unit C are not choosing to use the service, I use 'client' because this is how everyone in Unit C referred to residents at the time of my fieldwork.

Borderline personality disorder

Another important label (which had been applied to a number of women who participated in this research) is Borderline Personality Disorder (BPD). This is a controversial diagnosis as a disorder of the personality that has been historically described as untreatable. The associated characteristics constituting a Borderline Personality Disorder diagnosis are distinctly different than those found in other types of personality disorder criteria. These adapted from *The Diagnostic and Statistical Manual of Mental Disorders* (DSM-IV) include: 'a lack of self-identity, dissociative symptoms, intense affective instability including anger, anxiety, depression and tension, patterns of thought similar to transient 'psychotic' symptoms, difficulties with interpersonal relationships, impulsiveness, self-injury, eating disorders and substance misuse' (Stafford, 1999:7). In particular, the items relating to relationships are 'frantic efforts to avoid real or imagined abandonment', experiencing 'a pattern of unstable and intense interpersonal relationships characterized by alternating between extremes of idealization and devaluation' and 'inappropriate, intense anger or difficulty controlling anger (e.g., frequent displays of temper, constant anger, recurrent physical fights)' (American Psychiatric Association, 1994:654).

Feminist authors emphasise the ways the BPD diagnosis is figured as something a patient 'has', rather than how their behaviour has adapted over the course of their lives. A study by Shaw and Proctor claims that 75% of those diagnosed with BPD are women (Shaw and Proctor, 2005), leading them to believe that this diagnosis is constructed around gendered expectations. They say that the diagnosis of BPD:

> depends on a psychiatrist judging whether emotions are appropriate/healthy with reference to the norm of 'rationality.' This means that both anger and fear of abandonment can be – and frequently are – judged to be inappropriate, as opposed to being understandable in the context of a person's history of being violated or abandoned.
>
> (Shaw and Proctor, 2005:485)

Shaw and Proctor theorise that the BPD diagnosis is applied to women who do not conform to normative gender roles because of their expression of anger or aggression, and conversely it can also be given to women who conform too strongly, by internalising their anger and expressing it as self-harm. They point out that because the BPD diagnosis is more likely to apply to people with abusive pasts, terminology such as Post Traumatic Stress Disorder (PTSD) should be used, which although still referred to as a 'disorder', does provide some indication to the trauma experienced. They comment on the rise in prevalence of the diagnosis of BPD as opposed to PTSD, and say this represents:

> a shift from a limited recognition of the extent and impact of the trauma associated with sexual violence, to a widespread acceptance of an individualizing and pathologizing model of mental distress which conceals sexual abuse by focusing on categorizing, blaming and 'treating' the survivors.
>
> (Shaw and Proctor, 2005:487)

Wilkins and Warner (2001) describe this situation as perpetuated by the BPD diagnosis, when behaviour that is used to cope with distress and trauma becomes indicative of a disorder, and victims' anger and distress become silenced yet again.

As with the label 'learning disability', it is necessary to carefully explore the social construction and use of the BPD label. Whilst not all women on Unit C were diagnosed with BPD, as I have described elsewhere (Fish, 2000), these terms are commonly used to describe learning disabled women who self-harm, whether or not they have a formal diagnosis. I argue that the main issue here is that problems are being attributed to the individual women, rather than the situations and events that they have experienced throughout their lives. These events are related to inequalities brought about by gender, disability and social class, and are themes which recur throughout this book.

Unit C

The research site is an NHS learning disability forensic trust which offers 'assessment, treatment and rehabilitation' within secure environments, including medium and low secure, enhanced and 'step-down services' (supported houses in the grounds). The aim is to support people through their care pathway from admission to eventual discharge into community settings such as group homes. People are admitted for a number of reasons including prison transfers, diversion from the Criminal Justice System (CJS), breakdown of previous placement or behaviour which is judged to put them at risk to themselves or others. Most of the clients have been through the CJS and have been assessed as suitable by the Community Learning Disabilities Team, or sectioned under the Mental Health Act (Department of Health, 2007b) due to a further diagnosis of mental disorder.

The unit had separate wards for women and men, but only approximately 20% of clients were women. They lived on single sex wards that contained between two and eight women. Clients received an individual care plan package, which included input from psychiatry and psychological treatment services, occupational therapy and specialist nursing support.

Historically, the unit was a traditional asylum which was built in 1914. From 1915 to 1920 it was designated as a 'military hospital' and treated 56,800 soldiers for wounds and sickness. Following the First World War, the hospital was returned to the Asylums Board and opened in 1921 to admit 'mental defectives'. When the British National Health Service was established in summer 1948, more than 2,000 people lived at the institution. There was a functioning farm, and an upholsterers where patients worked, as well as a huge auditorium with stage, shops and clubs (see also Bogdan and Marshall, 1997). Since the 1990s, in the context of the *National Health Service and Community Care Act* (1990), most of the large ward buildings have been demolished and purpose-built modern buildings have taken their place. Modern barriers guard the entrance to the grounds, yet the austere Victorian administration building, a symbol of the past, remains.

The policy context: the development of secure services for learning disabled people

From the 1900s until the late 1970s in the UK, offenders with learning disabilities and those at risk of offending were placed in institutions or high-secure hospitals. Provision of services for this group changed in the 1970s, after the publication of Nirje's (1969) principle of *Normalisation* (which I will discuss later), and the subsequent 1971 white paper *Better Services for the Mentally Handicapped* (Department of Health and Social Services, 1971) which introduced the government's intention to shift from institutional care to community care. This was part of wider government policy shift to provide community-based services for people with mental health conditions and physically impaired people who needed day-to-day support. During the 1980s and early 1990s, long-stay users were relocated to the community; the people who remained tended to be perceived as the most difficult to relocate (Mansell et al., 2007; Yacoub et al., 2008). For those who were unable to access the generic community services due to their 'clinical presentation', *The Glancy Report* (Department of Health and Social Services, 1974) and *The Butler Report* (Home Office and Department of Health and Social Services, 1973) advocated the creation of regional secure units in the NHS.

So although care in the community was the highest aspiration, it was recognised that some people who had broken the law and those who were considered difficult to manage within the community would need specialist residential services for rehabilitation. *The Reed Report* (Department of Health and Home Office, 1992) gave an overview of each 'group' of mentally disordered offenders and recommended that people be cared for in the least restrictive environment for their needs, as near to their home as possible. The report proposed that services should be designed with care and attention to individuals' needs, and as far as possible people should be cared for in the community, under no greater conditions of security than is justified, and in a way that promotes rehabilitation and chances of sustaining an independent life. Following this, *The Mansell Report* (Mansell,

1993), which related specifically to learning disabled people with complex needs, was published. Both of these reports emphasised the need for locally based secure services, reflecting the shift in views in response to activist movements, such as the Disability Rights Movement and the Independent Living Movement (Mansell et al., 2007).

Despite recommendations to place people as locally as possible, specialist services for learning disabled people have developed at varying rates, perhaps due to the small number of people requiring them. Consequently, placements may be hundreds of miles from home, which can present many difficulties such as loss of contact with local services and families (Stewart and Dakin, 2009). This was a current issue at the time of the study, as families were joining together to challenge the available service provision and the acceptability of the removal of their family member for reasons of 'challenging behaviour' (Ryan and Julian, 2015).

Women are particularly affected by the absence of appropriate provision, as some of these services are men-only, resulting in a higher probability of being placed far from home. *The Corston Report* (2007), which looked specifically at issues experienced by women in prison, recommended changing the way criminal justice agencies work with women, and replacing women's prisons with local custodial units as a way of addressing these issues. Some academic literature suggests that there is less of a need for high levels of physical security and more need for 'relational security' for the majority of women offenders (Hassell and Bartlett, 2001; Long et al., 2008). Relational security is defined by the Department of Health as 'the knowledge and understanding staff have of a patient and of the environment; and the translation of that information into appropriate responses and care' (Department of Health, 2010). Despite these recommendations, some researchers have demonstrated that women are detained within higher levels of security for less severe crimes than men, and certainly higher than is justified (see Bland et al., 1999).

Until 2007, there was a lack of nationally agreed standards in England and Wales for medium secure care, leading to confusion as to whether units were classed as medium or low secure. As a result of the growing private and voluntary sector provision, the Department of Health released *Best Practice Guidance: Specification for Adult Medium-Secure Services* (Department of Health, 2007a) which gave clear standards for service agreements. Nevertheless, there are still concerns that some people confined in these services are wrongly placed due to their behaviour being inappropriately treated as criminal, when there is no criminal intent (Douds and Bantwal, 2011).

An investigation into prisoners' needs commissioned by the Prison Reform Trust, *No One Knows* (Talbot and Riley, 2007) reported that a significant number of people in prison could be described as learning disabled due to their IQ scores. This flagged up concerns about the pathways to prison and the links between courts, prisons and learning disability teams. For this reason, *The Bradley Report* (Bradley, 2009), an independent review of people with mental health conditions and/or learning disabilities within the criminal justice system, was commissioned. This report set out a national strategy for better screening and more appropriate placement of these people, and rehabilitation services for this group. Although accessing the relevant service is important (Glaser and Deane, 1999), being placed in a specialist unit rather than prison means there is no release date, resulting in some people being confined for many years. Furthermore, women tend to spend longer in secure units due to their level of behavioural disturbance (Hayes, 2004). This situation has caused questions to be asked about whether such units are indeed better than prison for learning disabled people, and whether detaining them with no clear plan for release infringes their human rights (Hayes, 2007).

It is clear that this type of service is still evolving in policy terms. Provision for offenders with learning disabilities, in particular for women, is evidently not ideal. The flaws in the diversion system means that some people are inappropriately sent to prison, where discrimination and bullying is prevalent (Talbot and Riley, 2007). Although policy is slowly responding to this concern, and more and more women are being diverted away from the prison system, the question asked by *The Corston Report* (2007) remains – why are women as a minority group residing in services that are largely designed around the needs of men?

Transforming care?

In 2011 the BBC broadcast a Panorama programme called *Undercover Care: The Abuse Exposed*. It showed hidden camera footage which depicted staff abusing people with learning disabilities at Winterbourne View, a private inpatient unit for people with learning disabilities and autism in Hambrook, South Gloucestershire. In response to the programme, staff members were put in prison and the hospital was closed down. The Department of Health commissioned a report called *Transforming Care: A National Response to Winterbourne View Hospital* (2012), which made an action plan to close inpatient units and move people back to their communities. The strategy was to find out how many people were in units because of challenging behaviour, for those detained to have better plans and for units to be safer.

Then, in 2014, a further report called *Winterbourne View – Time for Change* was released. The report said that people with learning disabilities and their families should have more power and support. This report made 11 suggestions, which were published in a plan called *Building the right support* in 2015. This discussed the need for good community services so people could move out of units. It set targets to cut down the amount of people in units by about half before 2019, and specified that people who have been in hospital or units for more than 5 years should be moved to the community first. Despite these several steps in the right direction, around 3,500 people remain in UK inpatient placements (Hatton, 2016).

General learning disability policy in the UK

Articulated by Nirje (1969) and then adopted by US scholar Wolfensberger, the 'Normalization Principle' aimed towards 'eliciting and maintaining culturally normative behaviour and using culturally normative means to this end'

(Wolfensberger, 1970:291). Learning disabled people were expected to live in family type groups, experiencing life as near to 'normal' as possible. The normalisation movement was undeniably pivotal in changing lives for learning disabled people, strengthening the move towards deinstitutionalisation and community-based services (Mansell and Ericsson, 1996). Although the normalisation concept has since been criticised for reproducing inequality by advocating that people should fit in with a professionally designated view of 'normality' (Williams and Nind, 1999; Moser, 2000), many services continued to use normalisation as a prevailing ideology (Deeley, 2002).

The evolution of Person Centred Planning (PCP), the central principle of the 2001 White Paper *Valuing People*, moved away from normalisation with a focus on services, offering them something to work towards (Robertson et al., 2005). PCP is rooted in the principles of shared power and self-determination, encouraging learning disabled people and their families to be involved in the plans for their future (Sanderson, 2000). PCP, if performed correctly, should focus on capabilities rather than deficits, and reflect what is possible rather than what is available (Sanderson, 2000). Although this sounds like a positive step in moving services forward, some authors claim that services are not following the principles correctly due to underfunding (Beresford, 2014), and others maintain that PCP remains a largely paper-based exercise (Mansell and Beadle-Brown, 2004). Indeed, some people, including those with mental health needs, are less likely to receive or benefit from person centred planning (Robertson et al., 2007).

Valuing People Now (2009), a new three-year strategy, reiterated the central recommendations of *Valuing People*, that learning disabled people have the same rights as everyone else, and are entitled to independent living, control and inclusion. Although these white papers focus on a person-centred agenda, criticisms have concentrated on the use of the neoliberal concepts of 'choice' without altering the system architecture to facilitate real control and inclusion (Kendall, 2004; Burton and Kagan, 2006). Indeed, according to Kendall, neoliberalist ideology now pervades policy and services for learning disabled people, as the preoccupation with the term 'choice' can mask the fact that opportunities are often narrow and constrained, and when there is perceived choice, individuals can be blamed for not taking the 'correct' path (Kendall, 2004).

In light of these claims, it has been argued that there is a discrepancy between white papers and policy for learning disabled people and the experience of people who use the services (Hollomotz, 2014). Adding to the knowledge-base of personal experiences of living in these services is essential. I hope to address this with my research, now and in the future.

My ethnographic methods

Locked wards have interested academics in social science for decades, but attention has largely been placed on psychiatric institutions rather than those specifically for learning disabled people. (Meehan et al., 2000; Meehan et al., 2004; Haw et al., 2011; Wadeson and Carpenter, 1976; Binder and McCoy, 1983; Hammill et al.,

1989; Goffman, 1961; Foucault, 1988; Bartlett, 2015). This book breaks new ground in applying ethnographic methods to a contemporary learning disability institution.

The ethnographic method I used was informed by feminist and disability studies principles. Both of these research traditions privilege the voices of marginalised groups and identify structural and societal barriers as the sources of inequality. While early disability scholars such as Finkelstein (1996) claimed that disability research should only centre on the structural barriers that cause disability, and questioned whether researching people's experience should be a valid focus for research (something that has been referred to as 'personal tragedy' modelling), Walmsley and Johnson (2003) point out that life history and ethnographic research traditions have led the field in inclusive learning disability research (Walmsley and Johnson, 2003). They argue that:

> disability studies and feminism have passed through the stage where narrating pain and oppression is what it is all about. However, just because others have done so does not necessarily mean that learning disability research will follow the pattern. Learning disabled people can contribute in many ways to research on situations where they possess unique and valuable experience. But to argue that they have the expertise to carry out or control all aspects of research is to go beyond the realms of the rational into a world where the reality of intellectual impairment is wished away and difference is denied.
>
> (Walmsley and Johnson, 2003:187)

Walmsley and Johnson therefore oppose the traditional view that learning disabled people are incapable of contributing to research. This comes from an idea put forward by Sigelman et al. (1981) in their oft-cited study about acquiescence. Here, it was claimed that learning disabled respondents provide ambiguous responses to interview questions. Although this work has been harshly critiqued (Hollomotz, 2017; Rapley and Antaki, 1996; Hutcheon et al., 2017), it continues to be cited in research articles. To challenge this, Walmsley and Johnson use examples of empirical research with learning disabled people that show how successful contribution is possible. Nevertheless, they also acknowledge difference in the form of 'impairment effects' (Thomas, 1999), which need to be taken into account in order to make the research process workable. This was an important implication for my research, showing the significance of following the guidance of disability and feminist studies in research with learning disabled people.

The women who participated in the research for this book were all labelled as having mild/moderate learning disabilities prior to admittance and were able to give consent. During the fieldwork, I observed the daily life of three of the flats where women were housed. Two of the wards were classified as low secure (LSU – wards are locked but clients are able to access other areas of the unit) and one was part of the medium secure unit (MSU – wards are locked, clients must stay within the two-storey, 5.2 metre enclosure at all times). I subsequently interviewed 16 clients from those wards and 10 staff from all areas of the unit, as a follow up to the observations.

I spent over 120 hours observing the life on the wards at different times of the day, over a period of nine months. Observations carried on during the interview phase and the whole of my fieldwork lasted 11 months altogether. My time on the wards involved much sitting and talking; many of the women said they were happy to have someone to talk to who did not have the duties of other staff. I purposefully did not spend too much time talking with staff on the wards, so that the women would not consider me to have a supervisory role. After two months of observations, I began asking people to take part in interviews. Prior to this research, I had been part of the Women's Action Group (WAG – a service user support group) for 12 months, so I knew many of the women and staff beforehand. I continued to be a member of the WAG whilst the research was ongoing. The group consisted of 10 women clients and their staff, and we met every fortnight for two hours to discuss issues relevant to women living on the unit, as well as organising social and fundraising events.

The women who knew me through the observational period and through my membership of the WAG group were much more likely to talk in-depth than women with whom I had little contact. One woman, for example, agreed to be interviewed but started to feel anxious and stopped the interview after about eight minutes. This woman was somebody with whom I hadn't had much contact and I was concerned about how the interview progressed. Most of the clients were very happy to talk in an interview, especially during times of little activity such as early evening or just before the evening meal. On the other hand, staff in both areas were difficult to pin down to be interviewed. There was often too few staff to allow one to leave the ward, or go to a separate room, and asking staff to be interviewed during their hard-earned break or after a 13-hour shift seemed excessive.

I visited each of the wards (which incorporated two flats, or apartments) during one day per week at different times to observe daily life there. I found this 'getting to know each other' period to be invaluable in gaining both clients' and staff's trust and subsequently, meaningful interviews; however, I was constantly wary of the ethical aspects and power imbalances in the research relationship. I found that spending time with people allowed me to explain the research project in much more detail to participants who might not easily understand its complexities.

Building friendships was difficult to avoid. There were a few instances where one of the clients 'took me under her wing' and I spent more time with some of the women rather than others. I do feel that I built a rapport with most of the participants, as I was often called upon to help out by escorting people to different places such as day services and 'women's hour', making drinks and unlocking doors which allowed me to spend time with different people; in fact at one point I was asked by the ward manager to provide an information session about mouth cancer during a 'community meeting' to help out. Many of the staff were aware of my previous research, and I was concerned that they would think that I was mainly observing them. I was always careful not to exploit the relationships I had built up, and kept in mind that my main research objective was to make recommendations which could improve the lives of women clients and staff on the wards.

Physically entering the wards was difficult. Each time I went to the low secure wards, I had to ring a bell to have the door clicked open remotely, and then someone had to come and unlock the internal doors with a key to let me in. I often had to explain about the research to a different person on the desk and was usually asked who I wanted to see. On the medium secure unit, I had to wait to enter a 'bubble': a space contained by two locked doors which cannot both be unlocked together. Then I had to give a key card with my identification on it through a hatch which looks like a bank till. In return, I got a belt with a pouch containing a bunch of keys on a nylon webbing strap and an electronic fob to unlock certain doors and a personal alarm. After organising these items onto the belt and pouch, I was let through into the MSU.

It was easier for me to move around the Medium Secure Unit. Having keys allowed me to access different areas and take clients to a range of rooms, including day services. Staff had been briefed about my visits and took the time to read the information sheets and help explain to clients my reasons for being there.

Spending time on the wards was enjoyable, but also distressing, intense and sometimes daunting. I had some fun with the clients and staff, but seeing people feeling angry, spending time with weeping women who had just self-harmed and listening to some stories from people's pasts was extremely distressing. I was always aware of Stacey's (1988) comments about people's lives merely translating into research data, and when women told me about the bad times in their lives I asked them if I could include it in the research. Usually the answer was 'yes, as long as you take my name out.' I was worried about how I was going to represent the people in the unit. I didn't want to 'other' the women clients myself by reinforcing gender and disability norms, or represent the staff as aloof or cold-hearted. Representation of people is a big responsibility and one I didn't take lightly, but I do acknowledge that my subjectivity and past experiences will affect my interpretations and how I write about people. Certain material has been left out of the book because of my commitment to ethical research and writing.

After two months of observations I decided to begin asking people to take part in interviews. Observations carried on during the interview phase and the whole of my fieldwork lasted 11 months altogether. I set out on the interviews with some questions in mind to help me focus on the reasons for my research:

- How do clients and staff experience day-to-day life on the wards?
- What do women clients value about the service?
- How do women feel they are progressing through the service?
- How do women clients and staff experience and perceive the staff/client relationship in this environment?
- How do staff and clients experience physical intervention, seclusion and enhanced observation?

I began interviewing by using a research schedule with specific questions to ask, which addressed the research questions loosely. The recommendations from

Unit C's management that obliged me to explore the subjects of seclusion, special observations and physical intervention meant I was compelled to introduce these subjects even if participants did not. However, I soon found that the interviews flowed better if I asked one or two questions and then prompted the participants for further information, so that they were introducing the themes of the interview themselves. I found that many of the participants did this, and I would just probe further into each theme that I wanted to look at. For example, when a participant started to speak about seclusion or physical restraint, I would probe this, saying something like, 'So, you mentioned being put into seclusion, how did that feel?'

I found the interviews with clients to be very successful, with a few clients commenting how much they enjoyed being interviewed and how it was good to get things off their chest. They had much to say about the service and were very open and honest. I think this is due to the rapport I built up with clients during the WAG and the observations in the flats, which I acknowledge has been to the cost of any rapport with staff. Time spent with the staff would have been at the expense of spending time with the clients; my time on the flats was always limited. Nonetheless, I did observe many interactions between staff and clients as well as conduct interviews with staff. I do hope, therefore, that this research project will be to the benefit of both groups.

Many of the things I was told as a researcher were difficult to hear, and I felt privileged to be in the trusted situation that allowed this, but also conscious that I was using this trust as a way to advance my own career. Disengaging myself from the relationships that had been built up was difficult (Rogers, 2003) but was made easier by my leaving to take maternity leave. I subsequently provided summaries for staff and accessible reports for clients, and presentations about the research for the organisation. (For a fuller explanation of my methods and ethical considerations, please see the Appendix of this book.)

Book outline

In the next chapter I describe the writing and knowledge that exists about women with learning disabilities. I use the scholarship as a way to understand the social position of these women historically and in contemporary society. I will show that there has been little opportunity for learning disabled women to give their opinions of services that they receive. Encouragingly, some of the literature which includes voices of learning disabled women shows the resilience and resistance of women, where they do not passively accept the roles and identities offered to them. I will explore learning disabled women's experiences both of power and resistance, in the context of the intersection between gender and disability. It is important to understand that learning disabled women are more complex than traditional normative and institutional representations suggest, in order to more fully recognise the adversities they encounter day-to-day. Indeed, this is particularly meaningful for those who have been removed from society and have little or no opportunity to join together.

Chapter 3 presents an overview of Unit C and provides my own first impressions, along with those of clients and staff. I introduce the women who were involved in my research, privileging their voices and their perspectives on life. I describe women's views on the reasons why they are in the unit and on their overall life experiences leading to their detention. I explore their daily activities, in an attempt to give an idea of how it feels to spend time on the unit and to show how gender, disability and also social class permeate day-to-day life on Unit C.

Chapter 4 analyses the relationships on the wards, how they are discussed and regulated by the service, and how women manage to find space for positive relationships. I explore the different relationships held by women on the unit, relationships with staff, other clients, and family. Finally, I discuss sexual relationships and how they are conducted on the wards. The chapter proposes that policy goals of safeguarding and independence work against women's capacities to form and maintain successful relationships, yet despite this regulation, many positive relationships prevail.

Chapter 5 explores how 'difficult' and rule-breaking behaviour is dealt with at Unit C. Staff have a number of ways to discourage and deal with risky or dangerous behaviour, such as the use of 'special observation', removal of belongings, and physical intervention for those considered at risk of self-harm. In addition, emergency medication, physical restraint and seclusion are used to deal with aggression. Here, I explore these overt strategies for control, questioning how the use of coercion shapes the therapeutic relationship and the progression of women through the service. I also describe more covert strategies for control, such as the control of information and movement. Issues of control, seclusion and restraint raise important questions about the power relations within the therapeutic relationship, including strategies of resistance. Women in Unit C pointed out the unpleasantness of coercive methods for both staff and client perspectives, and they emphasised the damage it could do to relationships. There were many opportunities being missed for discussion and resolution of conflict.

Chapter 6 discusses conceptualisations of progression and futures. I argue that for the service to be seen as achieving its objectives as a therapeutic establishment, examples of women moving through, and ultimately out of, the service are essential. Women outline their perceptions of rehabilitation and progression in this chapter, such as success in arranged relationships and acceptance of the institutional regime in order to progress. The chapter demonstrates how important notions of the future are to women, and how these plans provide them with ways of achieving the criteria for progression. The women's personal notions of progression (such as being able to talk about the past) were sometimes at odds with that of the organisation. This chapter shows how service objectives overshadow personal objectives in terms of everyday life. The usefulness of a feminist intersectional analysis coupled with a Disability Studies perspective becomes evident in discussions of women's strong sense of future, which also reflects their realistic expectations relating to disability, gender and social class.

Chapter 7 summarises the themes of the research and outlines the implications for changes in service delivery for learning disabled women. For instance, in exploring ideas about how women progress through the service, I found myself asking what the purpose of the service was. In formal descriptions, the service is described as 'treatment' and 'rehabilitation' yet these descriptions are only meaningful if the objectives filter into day-to-day life. In my observations and interviews, talk about behavioural stability pervaded concepts of progression to the cost of ideas of personal goals, or treatment and rehabilitation. It was clear that women were accessing psychological therapy, yet support staff were not trained in counselling, sometimes leaving women at a loose end when returning from a therapy session. Likewise, the book demonstrates the complexity of recognising the past traumas of these women while at the same time planning for a positive future. A focus on women's pasts cannot occur at the expense of consideration about their futures, but women's experiences of abuse and violence are extremely important when it comes to therapy and treatment. The consequences of these events can be taken into account as long as women's strengths and future aspirations also feature in the conversation. Many more institutional, practice and policy changes are identified, particularly around coercive practices of behaviour management.

Bibliography

American Psychiatric Association. (1994). *DSM-IV® sourcebook*. Washington, D.C.: American Psychiatric Publication.

Bartlett, A. (2015). *Secure lives: The meaning and importance of culture in secure hospital care*. Oxford: Oxford University Press.

Beresford, P. (2014). *Personalisation*. Bristol: Policy Press.

Binder, R. L., & McCoy, S. M. (1983). A study of patients' attitudes toward placement in seclusion. *Psychiatric Services*, 34, 1052–1054.

Bland, J., Mezey, G., & Dolan, B. (1999). Special women, special needs: A descriptive study of female special hospital patients. *Journal of Forensic Psychiatry & Psychology*, 10, 34–45.

Bogdan, R., & Marshall, A. (1997). Views of the asylum: Picture postcard depictions of institutions for people with mental disorders in the early 20th century. *Visual Studies*, 12, 4–27.

Bradley, B. (2009). *The Bradley Report: Lord Bradley's review of people with mental health problems or learning disabilities in the criminal justice system: Executive summary*. London: Department of Health.

Brown, M., James, E., & Hatton, C. (2017). *A trade in people: The inpatient healthcare economy for people with learning disabilities and/or Autism Spectrum Disorder*. Lancaster: Centre for Disability Research.

Burton, M., & Kagan, C. (2006). Decoding valuing people. *Disability & Society*, 21, 299–313.

Chapman, M. (2011). Undercover care: The abuse exposed. *BBC Panorama*.

Corston, J. (2007). *The Corston Report: A report of a review of women with particular vulnerabilities in the criminal justice system*. London: Home Office.

Deeley, S. (2002). Professional ideology and learning disability: An analysis of internal conflict. *Disability & Society*, 17, 19–33.

Department of Health. (2007a). *Best practice guidance: Specifications for adult medium secure services: Health offender partnerships*. London: Department of Health.

Department of Health. (2007b). *Mental Health Act: Code of practice*. London: HMSO.

Department of Health. (2009). *Valuing people now: A new three year strategy.* London: Department of Health.

Department of Health. (2010). *See, think, act: Your guide to relational security.* London: Department of Health.

Department of Health. (2012). *Transforming care: A national response to Winterbourne View Hospital: Department of health review: Final report.* London: Department of Health. Available at www.gov.uk/government/uploads/system/uploads/attachment_data/file/213215/final-report.pdf (Accessed 18/07/2017)

Department of Health and Home Office. (1992). *Review of health and social services for people with learning disabilities and others requiring similar services: Final summary report (The Reed Report).* London: HMSO.

Department of Health and Social Services. (1971). *Better services for the mentally handicapped.* London: HMSO.

Department of Health and Social Services. (1974). *Revised report for the working party on security in NHS psychiatric hospitals (The Glancy Report).* London: DHSS.

Douds, F., & Bantwal, A. (2011). The "forensicisation" of challenging behaviour: The perils of people with learning disabilities and severe challenging behaviours being viewed as "forensic" patients. *Journal of Learning Disabilities and Offending Behaviour,* 2, 110–113.

Duperouzel, H., & Fish, R. (2010). Hurting no-one else's body but your own: People with intellectual disability who self injure in a forensic service. *Journal of Applied Research in Intellectual Disabilities,* 23, 606–615.

Finkelstein, V. (1996). Outside "inside out". *Coalition,* 2, 30–36.

Fish, R. (2000). Working with people who harm themselves in a forensic learning disability service: Experiences of direct care staff. *Journal of Learning Disabilities,* 4, 193.

Foucault, M. (1988). *Madness and civilization.* New York: Random House.

Gernsbacher, M. A. (2017). Editorial perspective: The use of person-first language in scholarly writing may accentuate stigma. *Journal of Child Psychology and Psychiatry,* 58, 859–861.

Gill, M. C. (2015). *Already doing it.* Minneapolis, MN: University of Minnesota Press.

Glaser, W., & Deane, K. (1999). Normalisation in an abnormal world: A study of prisoners with an intellectual disability. *International Journal of Offender Therapy and Comparative Criminology,* 43, 338–356.

Goffman, E. (1961). *Asylums: Essays on the social situation of mental patients and other inmates.* New York: Anchor Books, Doubleday & Co.

Hammill, K., Mcevoy, J. P., Koral, H., & Schneider, N. J. (1989). Hospitalized schizophrenic patient views about seclusion. *Journal of Clinical Psychiatry,* 50, 174–177.

Hassell, Y., & Bartlett, A. (2001). The changing climate for women patients in medium secure psychiatric units. *Psychiatric Bulletin,* 25, 340–342.

Hatton, C. (2016). Specialist inpatient services for people with learning disabilities across the four countries of the UK. *Tizard Learning Disability Review,* 21(4), 220–225.

Haw, C., Stubbs, J., Bickle, A., & Stewart, I. (2011). Coercive treatments in forensic psychiatry: A study of patients' experiences and preferences. *Journal of Forensic Psychiatry & Psychology,* 22, 564–585.

Hayes, S. (2004). Pathways for offenders with intellectual disabilities. In W. R. Lindsay, J. L. Taylor & P. Sturmey (Eds.), *Offenders with developmental disabilities* (pp. 68–89). London: John Wiley & Sons.

Hayes, S. (2007). Missing out: Offenders with learning disabilities and the criminal justice system. *British Journal of Learning Disabilities,* 35, 146–153.

Health and Social Care Information Centre. (2015). *Learning disability census report, England 30 September 2015 experimental statistics.* Leeds: HSCIC.

Hollomotz, A. (2014). Are we valuing people's choices now? Restrictions to mundane choices made by adults with learning difficulties. *British Journal of Social Work*, 44, 234–251.

Hollomotz, A. (2017). Successful interviews with people with intellectual disability. *Qualitative Research*, DOI: http1468794117713810 Available at http://journals.sagepub.com/doi/pdf/10.1177/1468794117713810 (Accessed 09/12/17).

Home Office and Department of Health and Social Services. (1973). *DHSS Report on the committee on mentally disordered offenders (The Butler Report)*. London: DHSS.

Hutcheon, E., Noshin, R., & Lashewicz, B. (2017). Interrogating "acquiescent" behavior of adults with developmental disabilities in interactions with caregiving family members: An instrumental case study. *Disability & Society*, 32, 344–357.

Jenkins, R. (1998). *Questions of competence: Culture, classification and intellectual disability*. Cambridge: Cambridge University Press.

Kendall, K. (2004). Female offenders or alleged offenders with developmental disabilities: A critical overview. In W. R. Lindsay, J. L. Taylor & P. Sturmey (Eds.), *Offenders with developmental disabilities* (pp. 265–288). Oxford: Wiley.

Long, C., Fulton, B., & Hollin, C. (2008). The development of a "best practice" service for women in a medium-secure psychiatric setting: Treatment components and evaluation. *Clinical Psychology and Psychotherapy*, 15, 304–319.

Mansell, J. (1993). *Services for people with learning disabilities and challenging behaviour or mental health needs: Report of a project group*. London: HMSO.

Mansell, J., & Beadle-Brown, J. (2004). Person-centred planning or person-centred action? Policy and practice in intellectual disability services. *Journal of Applied Research in Intellectual Disabilities*, 17, 1–9.

Mansell, J., & Ericsson, K. (1996). *Deinstitutionalization and community living: Intellectual disability services in Britain, Scandinavia and the USA*. London: Chapman and Hall.

Mansell, J., Knapp, M., Beadle-Brown, J., & Beecham, J. (2007). *Deinstitutionalisation and community living – outcomes and costs: Report of a European study: Volume 2: Main report*. Canterbury: University of Kent.

Mclaughlin, H. (2009). What's in a name: "Client", "patient", "customer", "consumer", "expert by experience", "service user" – what's next? *British Journal of Social Work*, 39, 1101–1117.

Meehan, T., Bergen, H., & Fjeldsoe, K. (2004). Staff and patient perceptions of seclusion: Has anything changed? *Journal of Advanced Nursing*, 47, 33–38.

Meehan, T., Vermeer, C., & Windsor, C. (2000). Patients' perceptions of seclusion: A qualitative investigation. *Journal of Advanced Nursing*, 31, 370–377.

Moser, I. (2000). Against normalisation: Subverting norms of ability and disability. *Science as Culture*, 9, 201–240.

National Health Service and Community Care Act. (1990). *Chapter 19*. London: The Stationery Office.

Nirje, B. (1969*). The normalization principle: Implications on normalization*. Symposium on normalization. Madrid: SIIS.

O'Brien, G. (2001). Defining learning disability: What place does intelligence testing have now? *Developmental Medicine & Child Neurology*, 43, 570–573.

Rapley, M. (2004). *The social construction of learning disability*. Cambridge: Cambridge University Press.

Rapley, M., & Antaki, C. (1996). A conversation analysis of the "acquiescence" of people with learning disabilities. *Journal of Community & Applied Social Psychology*, 6, 207–227.

Robertson, J., Emerson, E., Hatton, C., Elliott, J., Mcintosh, B., Swift, P. . . . Knapp, M. (2005). *The impact of person centred planning*. Lancashire, England: Lancaster University, Institute for Health Research.

Robertson, J., Emerson, E., Hatton, C., Elliott, J., Mcintosh, B., Swift, P. . . . Knapp, M. (2007). Person-centred planning: Factors associated with successful outcomes for people with intellectual disabilities. *Journal of Intellectual Disability Research*, 51, 232–243.

Rogers, C. (2003). The mother/researcher in blurred boundaries of a reflexive research process. *Auto/Biography*, 11, 47–54.

Ryan, S. (2017). *Justice for laughing boy: Connor Sparrowhawk – A death by indifference*. London: Jessica Kingsley.

Ryan, S., & Julian, G. (2015). *Actually improving care services for people with learning disabilities and challenging behaviour*. Oxford: JusticeforLB Herb Audit Office.

Sanderson, H. (2000). *Person-centred planning: Key features and approaches*. York: Joseph Rowntree Foundation.

Shaw, C., & Proctor, G. (2005). I: Women at the margins: A critique of the diagnosis of borderline personality disorder. *Feminism & Psychology*, 15, 483.

Sigelman, C. K., Budd, E. C., Spanhel, C. L., & Schoenrock, C. J. (1981). When in doubt, say yes: Acquiescence in interviews with mentally retarded persons. *Mental Retardation*, 19, 53–58.

Simpson, M. (1999). Bodies, brains, behaviour: The return of the three stooges in learning disability. In M. Corker & S. French (Eds.), *Disability discourse* (pp. 148–156). Buckingham: Open University Press.

Stacey, J. (1988). Can there be a feminist ethnography? *Women's Studies International Forum*, 11, 21–27.

Stafford, P. (1999). *Defining gender issues: Redefining women's services*. London: Women in Secure Hospitals (WISH).

Stewart, M., & Dakin, L. (2009). An introduction to policy and service provision in forensic learning disabilities. In E. Chaplin, J. Henry & S. Hardy (Eds.), *Working with people with learning disabilities and offending behaviour: A handbook* (pp. 19–49). Brighton: Pavilion.

Talbot, J., & Riley, C. (2007). No one knows: Offenders with learning difficulties and learning disabilities. *British Journal of Learning Disabilities*, 35, 154–161.

Thomas, C. (1999). *Female forms: Experiencing and understanding disability*. Buckingham: Open University Press.

Wadeson, H., & Carpenter, W. T. (1976). Impact of the seclusion room experience. *The Journal of Nervous and Mental Disease*, 163, 318–328.

Walmsley, J., & Johnson, K. (2003). *Inclusive research with people with learning disabilities: Past, present, and futures*. London: Jessica Kingsley.

Wilkins, T., & Warner, S. (2001). Women in special hospitals: Understanding the presenting behaviour of women diagnosed with borderline personality disorder. *Journal of Psychiatric and Mental Health Nursing*, 8, 289–297.

Williams, L., & Nind, M. (1999). Insiders or outsiders: Normalisation and women with learning difficulties. *Disability & Society*, 14, 659–672.

Wolfensberger, W. (1970). The principle of normalization and its implications to psychiatric services. *American Journal of Psychiatry*, 127, 291–297.

Yacoub, E., Hall, I., & Bernall, J. (2008). Secure in-patient services for people with learning disability: Is the market serving the user well? *Psychiatric Bulletin*, 32, 205–207.

2   Learning disabled women in secure services

There is a small but growing literature that has explored the experiences of learning disabled women; however, there is very little research with women who live in residential services (Allen et al., 2001; Crawford, 2001; Taggart et al., 2008). Brown (1996) suggests that the reason for this is that learning disability services have traditionally hidden behind a 'gender blind' approach (see also Scior, 2003). In this chapter I reflect on what is already known about learning disabled women's lives, both in community settings and in secure services. I consider the suggestion that learning disabled women in secure services have similar experiences and needs as women living in secure mental health services (James and Warner, 2005), and delve into some of the specific concerns which arise in the literature about women in services, such as self-harm and sexual abuse.

Considering the relatively large amount of published literature and personal accounts detailing women's experiences of residential *psychiatric* services in the UK and US (for example Pembroke, 1996; Vincent, 2008; Jamison, 2009; Duke, 2010; Kaysen, 2013; Kennedy and Fortune, 2014), the scarcity of work on learning disabled women living in contemporary services is notable. Some authors have included women in residential services as research participants as well as women in the community (McCarthy, 1999; Scior, 2003), and others, including myself, have focussed on women in secure services but explored only a particular aspect of their lives (Sequeira, 2001; Harker-Longton and Fish, 2002; Duperouzel and Fish, 2008; Duperouzel and Fish, 2010; Fitzgerald and Withers, 2011). I have found only one study that explores the experiences of women living on a locked ward (Johnson, 1998). Perhaps due to the heterogeneity and medicalisation of the population of adults who have been labelled as learning disabled, traditional research has concentrated on medical syndromes and service provision (Aspis, 2000b) and has, until recently, been presented in a gender-neutral way, with papers not specifying the sex of their participants.

Throughout history, learning disabled women have not been provided with the opportunity to fully participate in both private and public aspects of society. As Traustadóttir and Johnson (2000:16) describe:

> In the past many [learning disabled women] have been excluded from their families during childhood and have been prohibited from forming adult relationships or families of their own. They have often been excluded from

work or community involvement or their participation has been voluntary or unacknowledged.

Women with learning disabilities have had very little representation or influence in the UK women's or disability movements (Aspis, 1997), and their circumstances have been hidden or overlooked (Atkinson et al., 2000). Traustadóttir and Johnson (2000:11) write about their involvement with learning disabled women, and report that they felt:

> outraged by the failure of those around them to recognise them as women or to take into account their concerns and desires . . . their stated desires and needs were ignored by families and service providers while their gender (when it was acknowledged) was constructed as a problem and a threat.

Researchers looking at the history of learning disability claim that traditionally, learning disabled women have been treated as a threat to society because of the combination of their sex and their impairment, and that this belief is still held in society today (see for example Phillips, 2007; Carlson, 2009).

Historical perspectives – institutionalisation

The construction of learning disabled women as a problem and a threat dates back to the European Eugenics movement of the early 20th century and the emerging philosophy of institutional medicine. The focus on women tended to be in terms of the possible social threat they posed through their capacity to have children. The Mental Deficiency Acts of 1913 and 1927 in the UK reinforced the ideology of this era by creating a legal framework by which to label and detain people on the grounds of their 'handicap' or 'moral defectiveness'. This framework was gender specific, targeting unmarried mothers and disabled women (Thomson, 1992; Walmsley, 2000; Carlson, 2009). These 'feeble-minded women' were considered to be promiscuous, carriers of disease and highly fecund (Phillips, 2007). Engwall (2004:78) observes that 'Feeble-minded men were seen as problematic due to their assumed tendency to turn into criminals, feeble-minded women were threatening society through their sexuality' (Engwall, 2004:78).

For most of the 20th century, learning disabled people in the UK, US and the Nordic countries were detained in large institutions, placed in sex-segregated wards and denied access to the workplace, family life and parenthood (Mansell and Ericsson, 1996). Thomson (1992) shows that the *Mental Deficiency Act* (1913) targeted girls as a sexual problem and that once they were institutionalised they often stayed for life. The Act led to the separation of many thousands of people from their families in an attempt to curb what was seen as a threat to society, particularly by women who were widely regarded as the likely bearers of 'defective' offspring (Carlson, 2001). These women usually had to undergo forced hysterectomy due to these pervasive beliefs (McCarthy, 1999; Atkinson and Williams, 1990; Tilley et al., 2012).

Women entered the institutions as children, young women or later in life when caring relatives had died (Phillips, 2007). Kristina Engwall, in her study of 481 medical records detailing the daily lives of women in institutions in early 20th-century Sweden, found that women were encouraged not to put too much emphasis on an attractive appearance, but rather on hard work, obedience and being on time. Prohibition of marriage and sterilisation 'excluded women from sexuality and fertility' (Engwall, 2004:83), and staff encouraged women into helping roles such as cleaning the communal areas or caring for other patients or children. In spite of this, Atkinson and Walmsley (1995) present accounts of women who had lived in UK institutions and remember gaining satisfaction from their imposed and unpaid roles as carers for less able patients in the institution. They also found ways to have forbidden relationships. Atkinson and Walmsley conclude that:

> These accounts remind us that even in such outwardly unpropitious circumstances women can still retain a sense of themselves as more than just victims. They are capable of resistance because, it seems, they possess a personal identity which is at variance with the label others have placed on them.
> (Atkinson and Walmsley, 1995:223)

Despite the dreadfulness of the way women were treated, it is clear that they were not just passive recipients of the social norms and values at that time, any more than they are today; they found ways to resist oppression and show strength in the face of adversity (Barron, 2002).

During the time of institutionalisation from the turn of the 20th century until the 1960s, medical discourses that showed interest in issues affecting learning disabled women were restricted to a consideration of how identified 'syndromes' and 'disabilities' expressed themselves differently in men and women and how they affected women's sexuality (Carlson, 2009). Traustadóttir and Johnson (2000) argue that this allowed professionals to dehumanise learning disabled people and treat them as objects of knowledge.

Wolfensberger's model of normalisation (Wolfensberger and Nirje, 1972) and O'Brien's Five Accomplishments model (O'Brien et al., 1981) advanced awareness of the disadvantages of institutionalisation in the UK, and supported the community-based living approach for learning disabled people that we see in evidence today. However, normalisation has been criticised by many, most notably as reinforcing traditional gender roles which serve to maintain a woman's place as being in the home or in low paid work (Brown and Smith, 1992). Women living in community care are often forced to live with other people (including men), who they have not chosen to live with; are placed in situations which mimic 'family life'; and encouraged to fulfil normative roles of domesticity taking on the bulk of the housework (Williams and Nind, 1999).

Research with learning disabled women in the community

Three notable books stand out within feminist research with learning disabled women in the community. In a landmark book detailing women's narratives by

Atkinson et al. (2000) *Good Times, Bad Times: Women with Learning Difficulties Telling their Stories* the experiences and life stories of learning disabled women are presented. Within what the authors describe as emancipatory research (Zarb, 1992), learning disabled women wrote their own stories, using academics as facilitators. The women relate what matters to them – employment, relationships and family. Although many of the accounts are positive, there is an overriding theme which touches all accounts – the women convey that they have been treated differently to other people; their needs have been ignored in some way. For example, some women described being disbelieved when reporting sexual violence; others said they had not been supported to get the lifestyle that they wanted, or were not paid a proper wage for their work. Simone Aspis, a learning disabled academic who has written many papers about her experiences, has described similar experiences of paternalistic practices on behalf of the professionals she has encountered (Aspis, 2000a).

A book by Traustadóttir and Johnson (2000), *Women with Intellectual Disabilities: Finding a Place in the World* presents collaborative research with learning disabled women from eight different countries, covering issues such as how women deal with the death of parents, friendships, work and violence and abuse. The theory and approach used in both of these books is consistent with both feminist and disability studies' concern to allow women to speak for themselves about what they consider to be important.

Michelle McCarthy offers a profound insight into the sexuality of learning disabled women from England. Her book *Sexuality and Women with Learning Disabilities* (1999) does not present women's narratives, but quotes from exceptionally rich in-depth interviews from the 17 women who were taking part in a sex education group with McCarthy. The women described themselves as having very little choice or control over their sexual experiences, and experiencing little or no enjoyment in intimacy. This was the case with women living in the community as well as in residential services. A large proportion of the group had experienced sexual abuse and gender-based violence.

More recent research includes papers by Scior (2000, 2003), who interviewed five learning disabled women in the UK. Her discourse analysis describes women frequently having their freedom and choices severely curtailed by carers. Scior claims that the 'historical construction' of these women as childlike and dependent lives on in policy and practice, leaving no space for acknowledging strengths and responsibilities (Scior, 2003:790). She talks of the 'inequality based on gender and disability' that is 'mediated through structural factors, such as education, employment, living arrangements and financial status' (Scior, 2003:784) and that can result in exploitation and low self-esteem. Scior therefore reminds us that although policy discourse relating to learning disabilities sounds liberating, featuring words like 'choice', 'control' and 'inclusion' – we should not forget the continuing influence and power of pervasive negative constructions. These constructions influence how women are treated, and make it very difficult for learning disabled people to think of themselves as having choice and control. Moreover, Björnsdóttir and Traustadóttir (2010) propose that the inequality experienced by learning disabled women is due to the way disability intersects with other social factors such as gender and class, leading to marginalisation and exclusion. Importantly however, they point out that people can challenge and resist society's disabling mechanisms.

Phillips recounts the narratives of eight older learning disabled women from three locations in England, demonstrating how their bodies were central to their notions of self and, at times, their collective identities:

> Contemporary debate within Disability Studies has focused on the role of 'the body' in a social model understanding of disability and impairment. In this context, disability refers to the environmental and discriminatory barriers imposed by cultural and social situations, while the body is neglected and medicalised in relation to one's biological impairment. For people socially and medically labelled as having a 'learning disability' the reverse situation applies, whereby a perceived impairment of mind or intellectual ability extends to a perceived impairment of the body. Consequently for people with learning difficulties the body is a site of regulation by a range of welfare, educational and medical discourses and controlled by carers, parents and professionals.
>
> (Phillips, 2007:503)

Even though these women lived in the community, Phillips described them as feeling contained, organised and policed through a system of institutionalised discourses. Welfare and educational services decided where women should be housed and medical professionals and social workers surveyed and recorded every action: 'Case notes, daily logbook accounts, personal programme plans and reviews all document patterns of behaviour and personal bodily functions. Visits to the doctor, dentist, chiropodist, times of hair washing sessions, baths and personal hygiene recommendations are all noted' (Phillips, 2007:511). Weight, diet and food were high on the agenda in day centres, where women were weighed on a weekly basis, which Phillips interprets as centralising the female body form in the public arena. The women all felt that they had experienced a lack of choice over their dress and appearance, which they experienced as a form of control over their identity.

Roets et al. (2008), present a different side to the story. Rather than focussing on inequalities faced by learning disabled women, their ethnographical study of the life of Rosa, a self-advocate living in the community in Belgium whom they refer to as a 'femme fatale' with learning disabilities, centres on her strengths. Describing her as a strong, characterful woman, they challenge the construction of learning disability as a naturalised impairment. They argue that disability, like gender, is shaped and sustained by mechanisms of 'truth', power, and knowledge and they show how ideas about disability and gender can be contradicted. They portray Rosa's struggles as a mother and as a 'rebel' and attest that learning disability should not be an 'all-encompassing identity' (Roets et al., 2008:26). By focussing on Rosa's resistance to the dominant norms, they critique the essentialist notions of gender and disability and I follow this orientation in my study.

Learning disabled women in forensic services

Women are a minority in almost all medium secure units in England, with the exception of a few units specifically accommodating women (Byrt et al., 2001). Some women are described as having been admitted compulsorily for behaviours such as aggression or self-harm that were not classed as offences, or caused by mental disorders, but which opposed society's expectations of how women should behave (Byrt et al., 2001). Other women are admitted through the CJS diversion schemes operated by triage assessment at police stations or court; however, these have been described as under-resourced and lacking in proactive screening, and particularly inadequate with regard to links with learning disability services (Hunter et al., 2008). *The Bradley Report* calls for more consistent implementation of diversion policy in the CJS, better identification and assessment and for learning disability to be seen separately to mental illness (Bradley, 2009).

Most secure services have been set up with men in mind. *The Reed Report* comments that:

> In male dominated environments, women's needs including their more personal female needs are liable to be overlooked . . . Services need to be responsive and proactive in order to counteract these problems in order that women receive appropriate care, treatment, accommodation and rehabilitation with proper attention to their personal dignity.
>
> (Department of Health and Home Office, 1992)

Ifill (1998:14) agrees with this by claiming that 'female patients in a predominantly male setting do not always receive services that are geared to their needs . . . most provision is set up for the majority, in this case men.'

Most of the research about secure units has focused on the special hospital system, and Bartlett and Hassel (2001) comment that it would be difficult to know the extent to which findings in some parts of the health service would apply to other types of units. They suggest that women may be subjected to high levels of restriction not because of their own problems but because of the type of people who share the service with them:

> In small units, women may have no way of avoiding sexualised social contact with men who have a history of sexual and physical violence towards women. . . . The reluctance of some medium secure units to deal with women patients because of unsafe environments . . . may create further difficulty.
>
> (Bartlett and Hassell, 2001:306)

In her literature review about women offenders with learning disabilities, Hayes (2007) suggests that adequate diversity and local proximity of services for women is lacking. She recognises that despite some active interventions of those advocating on behalf of women, the justice system tends to remain male-focused and male-dominated and she recommends that further research to aid policy development is urgently needed. This would address the dearth of information in this area and enable the voice of women offenders with learning disabilities to be heard: 'Female offenders are a small, neglected and devalued group within the criminal justice system; the even smaller minority group with a learning disability have little in the way of specific resources, services or advocacy' (Hayes, 2007:190).

Crawford (2001) interviewed ten women with mild or borderline learning disabilities and staff in two secure units in England. The women were admitted to medium security as the result of damage to property, self-harming behaviour and aggressive behaviour displayed towards staff within less secure facilities. Seven of the women she interviewed had a diagnosis of personality disorder, five of whom had three or more diagnoses, including paranoid schizophrenia and 'emotional instability'. She reports that during admission 'all women had cut their bodies' (Crawford, 2001:6), and that 80% of women had attacked their carers and 70% had attacked their peers in the last year. Her interpretation was that the women used self-harm as a way to bring revenge upon their carers or to punish themselves. More commonly, however, women used self-harm as a way of releasing tension, a phenomenon also described in my own research (Fish and Duperouzel, 2008). Crawford describes the women as having developed a 'hierarchy' of self-harm, where the most dangerous acts would generate more response from staff; and she interprets this as the women ensuring she is not 'forgotten'.

With reference to gender identity, Crawford (2001) refers to an 'invisible gender' in secure services, which allows the service to ignore any potential differences between services offered to men and women. However, a woman's gender may become 'visible' due to her difficult behaviour, when the behaviour is blamed on her being a woman and a problem. Crawford reports one patient identifying her fears of losing her self-identity as a woman, due to the presence of male sex offenders on the unit, for example the service was limiting her leisure activities and the way she was allowed to dress (see also Fitzgerald and Withers, 2011). Crawford writes:

> The oppression of women as a visible gender allows for effective institutional functioning. Unsurprisingly, those who challenge the system are thought to be deviant and become a 'visible' hazard to the institution.
>
> (Crawford, 2001:156)

The evidence Crawford provides paints a picture of services as not having the means to recognise gender diversity or difference until it becomes a problem; this problem is then talked about as existing within the group of women, rather than being situational (see also Aiyegbusi, 2004). This type of discourse or language used about a person can affect their care; some studies show that behaviour that does not lie within gendered expectations is considered to be a sign of some pathology of the mind. Labels such as 'difficult' can be used by staff when talking about a person, and reinforced through case notes over long periods of time (Johnson and Webb, 1995; Peter, 2000; Williams et al., 2001). Crawford's paper points to discrete topics for potential research, but unfortunately does not offer any direct quotes from the transcripts to illustrate her interpretation.

Kelley Johnson's (1998) ethnographic research with learning disabled women living on a locked unit in Australia found that the perceptions surrounding these women had influenced the exclusion from their families and communities in the past. Johnson observed that the staff's ongoing descriptions of the women were privileged and fixed, which she explained as women's identities being constituted by the staff rather than the women themselves. She noticed that the sexuality of the women on the unit was either ignored, or talked about by staff in terms of either the threat of pregnancy or exploitation, rather than as an expression of desire (see also Barron, 2002). Staff saw themselves as primarily there to care for the women physically and though all of the staff commented that they took pride in caring for the women, they resented having to do so many household tasks. Due to the perceived shortage of time, special attention was given to some more 'difficult' individuals while others missed out. Staff made efforts to understand the women's 'challenging behaviour', sometimes seeing it as frustration over their living environment, and other times as 'attention seeking' or copying from the disruptive behaviour of other clients. Controlling aggression was seen by the staff as one of their most important functions or skills, but staff were restricted by the custodial nature of their relationships with the women.

As well as the clients, the staff were also described as being locked in. That is, there were few opportunities to go outside other than with a group of women for whom they were responsible. Johnson observed other shared experiences, most notably that the women were always under the surveillance of the staff and the staff were always watched by the women, something she refers to as a 'mutual gaze' which she describes as complex and ambivalent. Not surprisingly, relationships between the women were intimate, complex and confining, both within the group of staff and with the women who lived on the unit.

Johnson's findings reflect the struggle for control that staff experience with the women in their care, whilst themselves being subjected to controlling mechanisms and surveillance from the organisation. The staff wanted to have more time and scope to develop therapeutic relationships with the clients, but saw their roles as mainly custodial and (physical) health related. Areas which could have been explored with the women, for example sexuality, were avoided or construed as problematic. Johnson's findings are extremely relevant to the current study; however, due to the women clients on the unit not using speech for communication, she does not present any interview transcripts or experiences from the perspective of the women themselves. My study, whilst situated in a more contemporary institution, builds upon the work of Johnson and includes the voices of both the women service users and staff.

The institutional response to women in secure care

It has been noted for many years that mental health services are no different from other social institutions in having rules and practices that serve the interest of privilege. Hence, services are frequently responsible for compounding the past experiences of disempowerment of many clients rather than providing opportunities of acknowledgement, understanding and change.

(Williams et al., 2004:32)

According to Stafford (in a 1999 WISH publication), women in secure hospitals are more likely to be classified as having a personality disorder, to have experienced sexual and/or physical abuse (see also Lindsay et al., 2004) and to stay longer than men in secure care. Research indicates that women are involved in more incidents of aggression than men (Sequeira and Halstead, 2001; Alexander et al., 2006), are more likely to self-harm (Maden, 1996) and are construed by staff as more 'volatile' than men (Crawford, 2001). It is suggested that the institutional response to these complexities is to place women in services of higher security than needed (Berber and Boer, 2004), and that women who are detained in these services are problematised and pathologised without any recognition of the trauma involved in their pasts (Aitken and Noble, 2001; Brackenridge and Morrissey, 2010).

Furthermore, research has found that women in residential secure services are prescribed more psychoactive drugs than men, and in the case of sedatives and anti-depressants, five times more (Bartlett and Hassell, 2001; Powell, 2001). Women are often believed to contribute to staff stress and burn out due to the frequency of incidents of aggression and self-harm (Fish, 2000) and research within secure units suggests that staff and organisational responses to these types of incident are further distressing to women and viewed as punishments, for example the use of physical restraint and confiscation of belongings to control self-harm (Harker-Longton and Fish, 2002; Fish and Culshaw, 2005; James and Warner, 2005; Duperouzel and Fish, 2008; Duperouzel and Fish, 2010).

Aitken points out that a sense of 'unsafe uncertainty' is created by the discourse surrounding women in secure care, which perpetuates their powerlessness:

(W)omen patients become constructed as having particularly complex needs, being particularly challenging, and especially vulnerable to overt forms of abuse (all of course relative to men). Women are also constructed as 'too fragile' to be allowed to risk trying out therapies which explore the emotional and relational aspects of being, even at a woman's request. In effect, women are constructed as differently dangerous but more so than men – to services and to themselves. The consequence is that a culture of suppression of rage, anger, frustration, and fear is maintained, as is the communication of women's sense of vulnerability and powerlessness. Women are 'done to' rather than 'being with'.

(Aitken, 2006:727)

Women as 'done to' is abundant in the literature. Owen and colleagues, for example studied residential services for women with long-term mental health needs and found that staff felt that they knew what was best for the women, particularly around the care and treatment offered, as well as their sexuality and fertility. Frequent judgements were made concerning women's behaviour, particularly if it did not conform to social norms (Owen et al., 1998:286). Along similar lines, Kristiansen discusses the paternalism of services, in terms of an imposed form of 'diminished credibility' (Kristiansen, 2004:380) where women are not believed or trusted, and everything they do or say becomes interpreted as due to their impairment, or 'only to be expected'.

Learning disabled women are subjected to imposed views of staff and families about what they can do as well as what they can be. According to Scior (2003), learning disability literature and services often come across as 'gender blind', but gender and disability cannot be separated. Women in Scior's study generally took on board traditional essentialist conceptions of womanhood in order to be seen and accepted as women, for example by taking pride in the tasks of housework (also described by Burns, 1993). The pressure to conform to gender stereotypes is acknowledged by Phillips (2007) who claims that parents and staff members try to 'create and impress' an identity they desire onto women, for example by forcing them to dress as children (Phillips, 2007:508). Scior further suggests that women may be faced with contradictions and dilemmas within dominant discourses of gender and disability; and these contradictions are clear in other research, notably people's accounts of institutionalisation. For example, learning disabled women who were in asylums in the 1950s remembered being treated like children but also being given responsibility to look after less able people and children on the wards (Potts and Fido, 1991). Another example is the dilemma between dominant gendered conceptions of motherhood in society, and learning disabled women's descriptions of motherhood as negative (McCarthy, 1999; Scior, 2003; Björnsdóttir r et al, 2017), possibly used as a way to justify their exclusion from parenthood.

Issues relevant to women in secure services

As the literature suggests, there is a good case to be made that women in secure facilities may present different clinical challenges than men due to their previous experiences and different reasons for entering the service (Bartlett and Hassell, 2001; Sarkar and di Lustro, 2011). As I have suggested, it is possible that secure units are not meeting the needs of women as they represent a minority (Lloyd, 1995; Berber and Boer, 2004).

A number of themes are recurrent in the literature relevant to all women who are detained in secure services. A short overview of each theme will be given in the following sections:

Gendered expectations

Instead of special hospitals appealing to women as a source of help and support they consistently fail to offer constructive treatment and the fact that a convicted woman once admitted to a special hospital loses her release date and can be detained indefinitely causes women to fear transfer no matter how bad her prison experience is. In this context there appears to be considerable confusion throughout the criminal justice system about what to do about female deviance.

(Powell, 2001:2)

Authors have suggested that women are overrepresented in secure care (in comparison with prison) because of their gender: 'Because we feel differently about women committing crime, we go to great lengths to avoid defining them as criminal, preferring the idea that they have emotional problems; they are mad rather than bad' (Probyn, 1990 cited in Warner, 1996:113). Therefore, gender discourse and expectations play a crucial role in the labelling of female deviance (Lloyd, 1995; Powell, 2001).

Allen (1987) found that women appearing before court are twice as likely as men to be dealt with by psychiatric means, in that they are more likely to be referred for psychiatric report, more likely to be found 'insane' or of diminished responsibility and if convicted, more likely to be placed in a secure service in place of a penal sentence. Allen claimed that these findings cannot be explained by differences in the mental health of offenders, and suggests that they are connected to gendered expectations. Other writers point to the antecedents and the contextual nature of women's behaviour, for example Williams et al. (2004), drawing on interviews with staff in a secure mental health unit, propose:

> It is inappropriate to conceptualise women's mental health problems in terms of individual pathology. It is both more accurate and more useful to conceptualise women's mental health problems as responses to, and sometimes as creative ways of coping with, damaging experiences that are rooted in their lived experiences of inequality and abuses of power.
>
> (Williams et al., 2004:32)

They go on to say that 'psychiatric labels supplemented with ward-based jargon are the raw material of women's reputations. This information, together with details of their index offence, precedes them into all settings' (Williams et al., 2004:37). Although it could be argued that these experiences also apply to mental health conditions of men, in a different paper, Williams et al. (2001) show how the combination of structural inequality, lack of access to resources and processes of hiding injustice such as victim blaming, is particularly significant for women's mental health.

It seems that even at the point of admission, women are at a disadvantage within the forensic system. The worrying fact is that their release date is dependent on the opinions of the same professionals who admit them to the service.

Control or therapy?

Researchers writing about secure care recognise the contradictions that apply when working with the client group (Deeley, 2002; Moyle, 2003; Bowers, 2006). Owen

(1998) found that service providers appeared to experience a conflict between protecting the women from their perceived vulnerabilities, and respecting their rights, including the right to safety, privacy, choice, support and independence.

Wilkins and Warner (2001) discuss the conflict between positioning clients as vulnerable children and at the same time as adults responsible for their actions. Consequently, a contradiction arises regarding the treatment and security: security is demanded by society but treatment is essential in defining a hospital as an institution. It is suggested that the hospital then becomes anti-therapeutic, as tensions emerge between control and therapy. Powell asks: 'how can a woman patient trust the person they are talking to/being treated by when part of their job is to report on her and be her jailer?' (Powell, 2001:5).

Research at secure units reveals that the conflict between 'duty of care' and therapeutic risk is a significant concern for staff (Fish, 2000; Fish et al., 2012), and this conflict can affect and characterise relationships between staff and clients. As would be expected in a closed unit, relationships with staff are very important to clients (Harker-Longton and Fish, 2002; Fish and Duperouzel, 2008; Clarkson et al., 2009); however, they can be difficult to develop and are often frustrated by staff moves, high levels of long-term sickness and ward changes. Wilkins and Warner advocate that

> In order to facilitate and maintain a secure base for patients, staff also require a secure base. Time for reflection and formal emotional support, should be an essential daily aspect of the role of clinical staff, rather than in times of crisis.
>
> (Wilkins and Warner, 2003:36)

This concept of positive therapeutic relationships as providing a 'secure base' is a reflection of the clinical application of attachment theory (Bowlby, 1977, 2005), which proposes that the types of bonds made during early life have a long-term effect on interpersonal relationship dynamics. In the absence of developing secure relationships, these relational patterns are in danger of recurrence. The use of attachment theory is particularly relevant to women's relationships and recurs throughout my work. In this book, I will show the importance of supporting and protecting secure relationships.

Self-harm

Self-harm in secure units has been found to be prevalent for both men and women (Burrow, 1992) and people who repeatedly self-harm have been described as one of the most challenging groups of patients (Huband and Tantam, 2000). Self-harm in the non-learning disabled population is primarily defined as intentional harm to one's own body without conscious suicidal intent, and may involve cutting, self-poisoning, ingesting objects, self-neglect, burning and breaking bones. These forms of self-harm have been described by people diagnosed with mild/moderate learning disabilities in terms of a way of coping, a symptom or disclosure of distress, a physical release from frustration, or a form of self-punishment (Harker-Longton and Fish, 2002; James and Warner, 2005).

As I have reported elsewhere, learning disabled people have stated that their self-harming behaviour is helpful to them at times of emotional strain (Duperouzel and Fish, 2008; Duperouzel and Fish, 2010). Clients did not feel they should be prevented from hurting themselves, and described how this organisational response was in fact contributing to their distress and ultimately maintaining their self-harm (Duperouzel and Fish, 2010). However, intentional damage to the body seems to be an extremely difficult form of expression for health professionals to process and deal with (Babiker and Arnold, 1997; Fish and Reid, 2011). This may be because nursing staff can experience working with people who self-harm to be challenging and draining, becoming frustrated when they don't see a decrease in self-harming behaviour over time (Fish, 2000).

Warner and Wilkins propose that women use self-harm as a coping behaviour in the absence of any alternative, because expressions of extreme anger and distress in any other form are discouraged for women:

> Turning rage and depression inwards may have less to do with women's biological inadequacies and more to do with their social marginalisation and subjugation. We should be careful, therefore, not to pathologise individuals for what might be better understood as being the result of social inequality and restricted choice.
>
> (Warner and Wilkins, 2004:267)

Incarcerating a person due to their self-harm is certainly a way of pathologising their behaviour, and is mainly rationalised as for reasons of safety. Learning disabled women may be particularly susceptible to this intervention, as the label of learning disability may conceal similarities and exaggerate differences between them and non-disabled women (James and Warner, 2005); in other words, the self-harm may be attributed to their impairment rather than their experiences. A small number of studies have looked at understandings of self-harm from the point of view of women with learning disabilities in the UK. James and Warner's (2005) study concluded that controlling women using restrictive methods traditionally used with male offenders would be to additionally penalise them and maintain their self-harming behaviour. The patients and staff in their research described using self-harm as a coping strategy to deal with past traumatic experiences, current relationships and issues around privation and security.

The incorporation of self-harm into an individual's life can be a gradual process in which self-harm increases in meaning to the person over time (Lovell, 2008). Harker-Longton and Fish's (2002) in-depth case study of Catherine, one woman with learning disability who self-harmed, found that this behaviour can provide many meanings and functions, such as feelings of euphoria, release of frustration and self-punishment. Catherine described her scars as emblems of past distress. The service's response to her self-harm was prevention, and sometimes seclusion, which served to make her feel punished. Catherine was insistent about preferring female staff who cared and understood about self-harm.

Functions described by Catherine such as self-punishment, communication of frustration and rebellion are recognised by Burstow (2004) who also acknowledges the addictive high that Catherine described as a 'wide awake' feeling (Harker-Longton and Fish, 2002:143). Liebling et al. (1997) and McCarthy (1998) discuss the struggle for control and power for women using services, which was also present in Catherine's account. Self-harm is argued by many feminist writers to be a response to distressing experiences in childhood (James and Warner, 2005), and this has been corroborated with empirical research, as childhood sexual and physical abuse, neglect, and childhood separation and loss have all been implicated (Gratz, 2003).

Sexual violence

Learning disabled women have been described as facing double oppression at the intersection of gender and disability, and this oppression makes them particularly vulnerable to sexual violence and exploitation (Brown, 2004). Early attempts to communicate abuse are often not believed, and even when abuse is disclosed in adulthood this can be ignored by services (Wilkins and Warner, 2003). Frequently, when women are offered support it is not the right kind (Atkinson et al., 2000; Traustadóttir and Johnson, 2000).

Adshead (1994) examined women's referrals to a forensic service. She found that 81% reported childhood sexual abuse, mainly by perpetrators known to the woman, and a further 56% had experienced sexual assault during adulthood. Most of the women had been diagnosed with Personality Disorder (66%), with 44% specified as having Borderline Personality Disorder, and all women had committed at least one act of self-harm with 87% regularly harming themselves.

Childhood abuse has been connected with the label of Borderline Personality Disorder (BPD). As I have said, this is a very common diagnosis for women who are detained in secure services, particularly secure mental health or learning disability services. Wilkins and Warner explored the connection between childhood abuse and this diagnosis. They concluded from interviews with staff that staff 'perceive relationships as an internalised difficulty for these women', and point out that 'problems are associated with abuse, abuse is internalised as a problem for women, therefore women and problems becomes connected – women are then condemned as essentially problematic' (Wilkins and Warner, 2003:33–34). Warner proposes that services construct these past difficulties as part of personality, rather than socially situated and relational (Warner, 1996). Other literature demonstrates how women with past abuse are perceived. Mansell et al. (1998), for example, propose a link between abuse and offending in later life, and indeed the knowledge of past abuse is claimed to increase risk categorisation in services (Pollack, 2007).

Aggression

Sequeira and Halstead (2001) found that learning disabled women in a residential service were involved in a disproportionately high number of aggressive incidents that had resulted in seclusion, restraint or tranquilisation. They also found that women had a significantly higher probability of being given rapid tranquilisation following a violent incident. In earlier research (Fish and Culshaw, 2005), I report on interviews with staff and clients at a medium secure unit about their experiences of aggressive incidents. Women clients reported that physical restraint, the most commonly used intervention at the unit, could trigger memories of abuse they had suffered in the past, particularly if a male staff member was involved. Some of the clients felt that physical restraint was being used as a punishment rather than as a 'last resort' measure, and all of the participants (including staff) gave negative comments about the use of physical restraint at the service.

Conclusion

Existing literature demonstrates that the experiences of women who become detained in secure learning disability services are complex and may be different to those of men due to their life experiences of gender-based marginalisation and discrimination (Sarkar and di Lustro, 2011). It has been suggested by many sources that women are not being placed appropriately in services which are designed for male offenders, and that the level of security in these services is inappropriately high for many women, who should be treated more therapeutically in smaller community-based units (Lindsay and Taylor, 2005; Benton and Roy, 2008; Wootton and Maden, 2010; Sarkar and di Lustro, 2011; Powell, 2001). This type of unit is being established in some areas of the UK (Wootton and Maden, 2010) and their remit is to provide more accessible locally based services, with high levels of therapy in a non-oppressive environment. Yet, large secure services where women are kept far from home, often for many years, prevail.

When women are incarcerated within secure services, a lack of gender awareness and restrictive gender norms can contribute to the development of challenging behaviour and to difficulties in identifying the needs expressed through these behaviours (Clements et al., 1995). Women in medium secure services who repeatedly act out are subject to pejorative labels such as 'attention seeker' or 'manipulative', and these kinds of descriptions can endure for long periods of time, as I will show. The literature I have summarised in this chapter describes services trying to dominate, judge and control women for whom power, violence and gender are likely to have been historically connected (Bartlett and Hassell, 2001). The social and interpersonal context of individual behaviours is ignored, and therefore diagnostic systems disguise the way that women's 'deviance' is a product of its particular time or place (Marecek, 2006). This could be comprehended as part of a larger issue relating to the way women, in particular learning disabled women, are treated in society.

Services have been described as rationalising the degree of surveillance of women by labelling them as 'vulnerable', further emphasising their dependency on others for care and protection (Crawford, 2001; Hollomotz, 2009). Despite this, there is evidence that clients are not safe from harm and have suffered sexual violence from men who share their unit (Mezey et al., 2005), as I will also show in this study.

Within secure services, staff can assume instructional or controlling roles (Barron, 2002; McCorkell, 2011; McCabe, 1996) which neither they nor the women find effective for therapeutic care and relationships. Often, services encourage independence and self-sufficiency, as recommended by policy, rather than interdependence and supportive relationships which are valued by many women (Clements et al., 1995). More worryingly, clients can perceive organisational responses such as physical restraint and seclusion as punishment or even become retraumatised – remembering distressing events from their pasts which caused them to feel powerless (Sequeira and Halstead, 2001; Fish and Culshaw, 2005). These issues may be more relevant to learning disabled women because of their experiences as part of a multiply marginalised group, and as this literature review demonstrates, judged in contradictory ways as 'deviant' or 'dangerous' on one hand and 'vulnerable' and 'childlike' on the other.

This review of the available literature shows that there has been little opportunity for learning disabled women to give their opinions of services that they receive; they have been expected to tolerate and endure the marginalisation they have experienced. Encouragingly, however, much of the literature which includes *voices* of learning disabled women shows the resilience and resistance of women albeit on an individual rather than collective level. Women do not passively accept the roles and restrictive identities offered to them, and make attempts to show that they are also in control (Atkinson et al., 2006; Atkinson and Walmsley, 1995; Gillman et al., 1997; Goodley and Moore, 2000; Mitchell et al., 2006). It is important that research continues to reflect learning disabled women in this accurate way, and to make known the adversities they encounter day-to-day. Indeed, this is particularly important for those who have been removed from society and have little or no opportunity to collectivise and orchestrate their own representation.

Bibliography

Adshead, G. (1994). Damage: Trauma and violence in a sample of women referred to a forensic service. *Behavioral Sciences & the Law*, 12, 235–249.

Aitken, G. (2006). Women and secure settings. *Psychologist*, 19, 726.

Aitken, G., & Noble, K. (2001). Violence and violation: women and secure settings. *Feminist review*, 68, 68–88.

Aiyegbusi, A. (2004). Thinking under fire: The challenge for forensic mental health nurses working with women in secure care. *Forensic Focus*, 27, 108–119.

Alexander, R., Crouch, K., Halstead, S., & Piachaud, J. (2006). Long term outcome from a medium secure service for people with intellectual disability. *Journal of Intellectual Disability Research*, 50, 305–315.

Allen, H. (1987). *Justice unbalanced: Gender, psychiatry and judicial decisions*. Bristol: Open University Press.

Allen, R., Lindsay, W., Macleod, F., & Smith, A. (2001). Treatment of women with intellectual disabilities who have been involved with the criminal justice system for reasons of aggression. *Journal of Applied Research in Intellectual Disabilities*, 14, 340–347.

Aspis, S. (1997). Self-advocacy for people with learning difficulties: Does it have a future? *Disability & Society*, 12, 647–654.

Aspis, S. (2000a). A disabled woman with learning disabilities fights back for her rights. In D. Atkinson, M. Mccarthy, J. Walmsley, M. Cooper, S. Rolph, S. Aspis, P. Barette, M. Coventry & G. Ferris (Eds.), *Good times, bad times: Women with learning difficulties telling their stories* (pp. 73–86). Kidderminster: BILD Publications.

Aspis, S. (2000b). Researching our history: Who is in charge. In L. Brigham, D. Atkinson, M. Jackson, S. Rolph & J. Walmsley (Eds.), *Crossing boundaries: Change and continuity in the history of learning disability* (pp. 1–6). Kidderminster: BILD Publications.

Atkinson, D., Cooper, M., & Ferris, G. (2006). Advocacy as resistance. In D. Mitchell, R. Traustadóttir, R. Chapman, L. Townson, N. Ingham & S. Ledger (Eds.), *Exploring experiences of advocacy by people with learning disabilities: Testimonies of resistance* (pp. 13–19). London: Jessica Kingsley.

Atkinson, D., Mccarthy, M., Walmsley, J., Cooper, M., Rolph, S., Aspis, S. . . . Ferris, G. (2000). *Good times, bad times: Women with learning difficulties telling their stories.* Kidderminster: BILD Publications.

Atkinson, D., & Walmsley, J. (1995). A woman's place? Issues of gender. In T. Philpot & L. Ward (Eds.), *Values and visions: Changing ideas in services for people with learning difficulties.* Oxford: Elsevier Health Sciences.

Atkinson, D., & Williams, F. (1990). *Know me as I am: An anthology of prose, poetry and art by people with learning difficulties.* London: Hodder & Stoughton in association with the Open University.

Babiker, G., & Arnold, L. (1997). *The language of injury: Comprehending self-mutilation.* Hoboken, NJ: Wiley-Blackwell.

Barron, K. (2002). Who am I? Women with learning difficulties (re) constructing their self-identity. *Scandinavian Journal of Disability Research*, 4, 58–79.

Bartlett, A., & Hassell, Y. (2001). Do women need special secure services? *Advances in Psychiatric Treatment*, 7, 302–309.

Benton, C., & Roy, A. (2008). The first three years of a community forensic service for people with a learning disability. *The British Journal of Forensic Practice*, 10, 4–12.

Berber, E., & Boer, H. (2004). Development of a specialised forensic service for women with learning disability: The first three years. *The British Journal of Forensic Practice*, 6, 10–20.

Björnsdóttir, K., Stefánsdóttir, A., & Valgerður Stefánsdóttir, G. (2017). People with intellectual disabilities negotiate autonomy, gender and sexuality. *Sexuality and Disability*, 35(3), 295–311.

Björnsdóttir, K., & Traustadóttir, R. (2010). Stuck in the land of disability? The intersection of learning difficulties, class, gender and religion. *Disability & Society*, 25, 49–62.

Bowers, L. (2006). On conflict, containment and the relationship between them. *Nursing Inquiry*, 13, 172–180.

Bowlby, J. (1977). The making and breaking of affectional bonds. I. Aetiology and psychopathology in the light of attachment theory. An expanded version of the Fiftieth Maudsley Lecture, delivered before the Royal College of Psychiatrists, 19 November 1976. *The British Journal of Psychiatry* 130(3), 201–210.

Bowlby, J. (2005). *A secure base: Clinical applications of attachment theory.* New York, Routledge.

Brackenridge, I., & Morrissey, C. (2010). Trauma and post-traumatic stress disorder (PTSD) in a high secure forensic learning disability population: Future directions for practice. *Advances in Mental Health and Intellectual Disabilities*, 4, 49–56.

Bradley, B. (2009). *The Bradley Report: Lord Bradley's review of people with mental health problems or learning disabilities in the criminal justice system: Executive summary.* London: Department of Health.

Brown, H. (1996). Ordinary women: Issues for women with learning disabilities. *British Journal of Learning Disabilities*, 24, 47–51.

Brown, H. (2004). A rights-based approach to abuse of women with learning disabilities. *Tizard Learning Disability Review*, 9, 41–44.

Brown, H., & Smith, H. (1992). *Normalisation: A reader for the nineties.* Abington: Routledge.

Burns, J. (1993). Invisible women-women who have learning disabilities. *The Psychologist*, 6, 102–104.

Burrow, S. (1992). The deliberate self harming behaviour of patients within a British special hospital. *Journal of Advanced Nursing*, 17, 138–148.

Burstow, B. (ed.) (2004). *Radical feminist therapy: Working in the context of violence.* London: Sage.

Byrt, R., Lomas, C., Gardinar, G., & Lewis, D. (2001). Working with women in secure environments. *Journal of Pscyhosocial Nursing and Mental Health Services*, 39, 42–50.

Carlson, L. (2001). Cognitive ableism and disability studies: Feminist reflections on the history of mental retardation. *Hypatia*, 16, 124–146.

Carlson, L. (2009). *The faces of intellectual disability: Philosophical reflections.* Bloomington, IN: Indiana University Press.

Clarkson, R., Murphy, G., Coldwell, J., & Dawson, D. (2009). What characteristics do service users with intellectual disability value in direct support staff within residential forensic services? *Journal of Intellectual and Developmental Disability*, 34, 283–289.

Clements, J., Clare, I., & Ezelle, L. (1995). Real men, real women, real lives? Gender issues in learning disabilities and challenging behaviour. *Disability & Society*, 10, 425–436.

Crawford, J. (2001). *The institutional hazard of being a visible woman.* The first international conference on the care and treatment of learning disabled offenders. Preston: UCLAN.

Deeley, S. (2002). Professional ideology and learning disability: An analysis of internal conflict. *Disability & Society*, 17, 19–33.

Department of Health and Home Office. (1992). *Review of health and social services for people with learning disabilities and others requiring similar services, Final summary report (The Reed Report).* London: HMSO.

Duke, P. (2010). *Brilliant madness: Living with manic depressive illness.* New York: Random House.

Duperouzel, H., & Fish, R. (2008). Why couldn't I stop her? Self injury: The views of staff and clients in a medium secure unit. *British Journal of Learning Disabilities*, 36, 59–65.

Duperouzel, H., & Fish, R. (2010). Hurting no-one else's body but your own: People with intellectual disability who self injure in a forensic service. *Journal of Applied Research in Intellectual Disabilities*, 23, 606–615.

Engwall, I. (2004). The implications of being diagnosed a feeble minded woman. In K. Kristiansen & R. Traustadóttir (Eds.), *Gender and disability research in the Nordic countries* (pp. 75–95). Lund: Studentlitteratur.

Fish, R. (2000). Working with people who harm themselves in a forensic learning disability service: Experiences of direct care staff. *Journal of Learning Disabilities*, 4, 193.

Fish, R., & Culshaw, E. (2005). The last resort? Staff and client perspectives on physical intervention. *Journal of Intellectual Disabilities*, 9, 93–107.

Fish, R., & Duperouzel, H. (2008). Just another day dealing with wounds: Self-injury and staff-client relationships. *Learning Disability Practice*, 11, 12–15.

Fish, R., & Reid, H. (2011). Working with self-harm: Accounts of two staff groups. *Journal of Learning Disabilities and Offending Behaviour*, 2, 152–158.

Fish, R., Woodward, S., & Duperouzel, H. (2012). "Change can only be a good thing": Staff views on the introduction of a harm minimisation policy in a forensic learning disability service. *British Journal of Learning Disabilities*, 40, 37–45.

Fitzgerald, C., & Withers, P. (2011). "I don't know what a proper woman means": What women with intellectual disabilities think about sex, sexuality and themselves. *British Journal of Learning Disabilities*, 41, 5–12.

Gillman, M., Swain, J., & Heyman, B. (1997). Life history or "case" history: The objectification of people with learning difficulties through the tyranny of professional discourses. *Disability & Society*, 12, 675–694.

Goodley, D., & Moore, M. (2000). Doing disability research: Activist lives and the academy. *Disability & Society*, 15, 861–882.

Gratz, K. L. (2003). Risk factors for and functions of deliberate self-harm: An empirical and conceptual review. *Clinical Psychology: Science and Practice*, 10, 192–205.

Harker-Longton, W., & Fish, R. (2002). "Cutting doesn't make you die": One woman's views on the treatment of her self-injurious behaviour. *Journal of Intellectual Disabilities*, 6, 137–151.

Hayes, S. (2007). Women with learning disabilities who offend: What do we know? *British Journal of Learning Disabilities*, 35, 187–191.

Hollomotz, A. (2009). Beyond "vulnerability": An ecological model approach to conceptualizing risk of sexual violence against people with learning difficulties. *British Journal of Social Work*, 39, 99–112.

Huband, N., & Tantam, D. (2000). Attitudes to self-injury within a group of mental health staff. *British Journal of Medical Psychology*, 73, 495–504.

Hunter, G., Boyce, I., & Smith, L. (2008). *Criminal justice liaison and diversion schemes: A focus on women offenders*. Mental Health Briefing. London: Nacro.

Ifill, C. (1998). One of a kind. *Nursing Times*, 94, 14–15.

James, M., & Warner, S. (2005). Coping with their lives – women, learning disabilities, self-harm and the secure unit: A Q-methodological study. *British Journal of Learning Disabilities*, 33, 120–127.

Jamison, K. R. (2009). *An unquiet mind: A memoir of moods and madness*. New York: Random House LLC.

Johnson, K. (1998). *Deinstitutionalising women: An ethnographic study of institutional closure*. Cambridge: Cambridge University Press.

Johnson, M., & Webb, C. (1995). Rediscovering unpopular patients: The concept of social judgement. *Journal of Advanced Nursing*, 21, 466–475.

Kaysen, S. (2013). *Girl, interrupted*. New York: Random House.

Kennedy, J., & Fortune, T. (2014). Women's experiences of being in an acute psychiatric unit: An occupational perspective. *British Journal of Occupational Therapy*, 77, 296–303.

Kristiansen, K. (2004). Madness, badness and sadness revisited: Ontology control in "mental health land". In K. Kristiansen & R. Traustadóttir (Eds.), *Gender and disability research in the Nordic countries* (pp. 365–393). Lund: Studentlitteratur.

Liebling, H., Chipchase, H., & Velangi, R. (1997). Why do women harm themselves? – Surviving special hospitals. *Feminism & Psychology*, 7, 427–435.

Lindsay, W., Smith, A., Quinn, K., Anderson, A., Smith, A., Allan, R., & Law, J. (2004). Women with intellectual disability who have offended: Characteristics and outcome. *Journal of Intellectual Disability Research*, 48, 580–590.

Lindsay, W., & Taylor, J. (2005). A selective review of research on offenders with developmental disabilities: Assessment and treatment. *Clinical Psychology & Psychotherapy*, 12, 201–214.

Lloyd, A. (1995). *Doubly deviant, doubly damned: Society's treatment of violent women*. London: Penguin Books.

Lovell, A. (2008). Learning disability against itself: The self-injury/self-harm conundrum. *British Journal of Learning Disabilities*, 36, 109–121.

Maden, T. (1996). *Women, prisons, and psychiatry: Mental disorder behind bars*. Oxford: Butterworth-Heinemann.

Mansell, J., & Ericsson, K. (1996). *Deinstitutionalization and community living: Intellectual Disability Services in Britain, Scandinavia and the USA*. London: Chapman and Hall.

Mansell, S., Sobsey, D., & Moskal, R. (1998). Clinical findings among sexually abused children with and without developmental disabilities. *Mental Retardation*, 36, 12–22.

Marecek, J. (2006). Social suffering, gender, and women's depression. In C. Keyes & S. Goodman (Eds.), *Women and depression: A handbook for the social, behavioral, and biomedical sciences* (pp. 283–308). Cambridge: Cambridge University Press.

Mccabe, J. (1996). Women in special hospitals and secure psychiatric containment. *Mental Health Review Journal*, 1, 28–30.

Mccarthy, M. (1998). Whose body is it anyway? Pressures and Control for women with learning disabilities. *Disability & Society*, 13, 557–574.

Mccarthy, M. (1999). *Sexuality and women with learning disabilities*. London: Jessica Kingsley Publishers.

Mccorkell, A. D. (2011). *Am I there yet? The views of people with learning disability on forensic community rehabilitation*. D.Clin.Psych. Thesis, University of Edinburgh.

Mezey, G., Hassell, Y., & Bartlett, A. (2005). Safety of women in mixed-sex and single-sex medium secure units: staff and patient perceptions. *The British Journal of Psychiatry*, 187, 579.

Mitchell, D., Traustadóttir, R., Chapman, R., Townson, L., Ingham, N., & Ledger, S. (2006). *Exploring experiences of advocacy by people with learning disabilities: Testimonies of resistance*. London: Jessica Kingsley.

Moyle, W. (2003). Nurse – patient relationship: A dichotomy of expectations. *International Journal of Mental Health Nursing*, 12, 103–109.

O'Brien, J., Tyne, A., & Values into Action (1981). *The principle of normalisation: A foundation for effective services*. London: Campaign for Mentally Handicapped People.

Owen, S., Repper, J., Perkins, R., & Robinson, J. (1998). An evaluation of services for women with long term mental health problems. *Journal of Psychiatric and Mental Health Nursing*, 5, 281–290.

Pembroke, L. R. (1996). *Self-harm perspectives from personal experience*. London: Chipmunkapublishing.

Peter, D. (2000). Dynamics of discourse: A case study illuminating power relations in mental retardation. *Mental Retardation*, 38, 354–362.

Phillips, D. (2007). Embodied narratives: Control, regulation and bodily resistance in the life course of older women with learning difficulties. *European Review of History – Revue européenne d'Histoire*, 14, 503–524.

Pollack, S. (2007). "I'm just not good in relationships": Victimization discourses and the gendered regulation of criminalized women. *Feminist Criminology*, 2, 158–174.

Potts, M., & Fido, R. (1991). *A fit person to be removed: Personal accounts of life in a mental deficiency institution*. Plymouth: Northcote House Publishers Ltd.

Powell, J. (2001). Women in British special hospitals: A sociological approach. *Journal of Social Sciences and Humanities*, 5, 1–14.

Roets, G., Reinaart, R., Adams, M., & Van Hove, G. (2008). Looking at lived experiences of self-advocacy through gendered eyes: Becoming femme fatale with/out "learning difficulties". *Gender and Education*, 20, 15–29.

Sarkar, J., & Di Lustro, M. (2011). Evolution of secure services for women in England. *Advances in Psychiatric Treatment*, 17, 323–331.

Scior, K. (2000). Women with learning disabilities: Gendered subjects after all? *Clinical Psychology Forum* 137, 6–10.

Scior, K. (2003). Using discourse analysis to study the experiences of women with learning disabilities. *Disability & Society*, 18, 779–795.

Sequeira, H. (2001). Women with intellectual disabilities: Finding a place in the world. *Journal of Applied Research in Intellectual Disabilities*, 14, 412–413.

Sequeira, H., & Halstead, S. (2001). Is it meant to hurt, is it? *Violence Against Women*, 7, 462–476.

Stafford, P. (1999). *Defining Gender Issues: redefining women's services*. London: Women in Secure Hospitals (WISH).

Taggart, L., Mcmillan, R., & Lawson, A. (2008). Women with and without intellectual disability and psychiatric disorders: An examination of the literature. *Journal of Intellectual Disabilities*, 12, 191–211.

Thomson, M. (1992). Sterilization, segregation and community care: Ideology and solutions to the problem of mental deficiency in inter-war Britain. *History of Psychiatry*, 3, 473.

Tilley, E., Walmsley, J., Earle, S., & Atkinson, D. (2012). "The silence is roaring": Sterilization, reproductive rights and women with intellectual disabilities. *Disability & Society*, 27, 413–426.

Traustadóttir, R., & Johnson, K. (2000). *Women with intellectual disabilities: Finding a place in the world*. London: Jessica Kingsley Publishers.

Vincent, N. (2008). *Voluntary madness: My year lost and found in the loony bin*. London: Penguin.

Walmsley, J. (2000). Women and the Mental Deficiency Act of 1913: Citizenship, sexuality and regulation. *British Journal of Learning Disabilities*, 28, 65–70.

Warner, S. (1996). *Visibly special? Women, child sexual abuse and special hospitals*. Aldershot: Avebury.

Warner, S., & Wilkins, T. (2004). Between subjugation and survival: Women, borderline personality disorder and high security mental hospitals. *Journal of Contemporary Psychotherapy*, 34, 265–278.

Wilkins, T., & Warner, S. (2001). Women in special hospitals: Understanding the presenting behaviour of women diagnosed with borderline personality disorder. *Journal of Psychiatric and Mental Health Nursing*, 8, 289–297.

Wilkins, T., & Warner, S. (2003). Understanding the therapeutic relationship – women diagnosed as borderline personality disordered. *The British Journal of Forensic Practice*, 2, 30–37.

Williams, J., Scott, S., & Bressingham, C. (2004). Dangerous journeys: Women's pathways into and through secure mental health services. In N. Jeffcote & T. Watson (Eds.), *Working therapeutically with women in secure mental health settings: Forensic Focus 27* (pp. 31–43). London: Jessica Kingsley Publishers.

Williams, J., Scott, S., & Waterhouse, S. (2001). Mental health services for "difficult" women: Reflections on some recent developments. *Feminist Review*, 68, 89–104.

Williams, L., & Nind, M. (1999). Insiders or outsiders: Normalisation and women with learning difficulties. *Disability & Society*, 14, 659–672.

Wolfensberger, W., & Nirje, B. (1972). *The principle of normalization in human services*. Toronto: National Institute on Mental Retardation.

Wootton, L., & Maden, A. (2010). Women in forensic institutions. In D. Kohen (Ed.), *Oxford Textbook of Women and Mental Health* (pp. 139–146). Oxford: Oxford University Press.

Zarb, G. (1992). On the road to Damascus: First steps towards changing the relations of disability research production. *Disability & Society*, 7, 125–138.

A version of this chapter has been published as:

Fish, R. (2013). Women who use secure services: Applying the literature to women with learning disabilities. *The Journal of Forensic Practice*, 15(3), 192–205. DOI: https://doi.org/10.1108/JFP-09-2012-0016

3   Life on the unit

Chapter 2 showed how secure services can be construed as 'gender blind' – not recognising gender until women's 'deviance' become visible. Services regulate and control women in particular ways to avoid these challenges. The following chapters will consider whether the issues described in the literature are relevant for women in Unit C. Here, I present an overview of Unit C and provide my own first impressions, along with those of clients and staff. I will introduce the people who were involved in my research and describe their daily activities, in an attempt to give an idea of how it feels to spend time on the unit and to show how gender, (dis)ability and class permeate day-to-day life on Unit C.

First impressions

Beginning my fieldwork was the first time I had visited the purpose-built wards of this particular Unit.[1] Any time I had spent previously had been on wards which were situated in the 'old institution' areas, red-brick buildings with tall windows and very high ceilings which were arranged as flats. I was interested to see what the newer wards were like. Here, my fieldnotes show my first impressions of the low secure unit (LSU):

> The low secure building was purpose-built in 2004. It is surrounded by lots of greenery, and is a single storey red-brick building with windows that reach from floor to ceiling. There are 7ft high green railings surrounding the outdoor spaces, and separating external areas of each flat.
>
> A staff member, Denise, shows me round. We enter the building using a key code for the front door, other doors leading to flats are locked with keys. The entrance leads to a central reception area that consists of a long desk behind which staff are using computers and looking at diaries. Four flats lead off from corridors away from the reception, but there are various doors that are visible from reception, some of which are meeting rooms which are being used as offices. Also visible from this area is the entrance to the seclusion area with its glass window.
>
> Entering the flat, there is an archway leading to the empty lounge that is neither clinical nor homely in atmosphere. The carpets are thin and hard,

there are no books, games, blankets or personal items strewn about. It is almost corridor-like, with furniture along the walls and a patio style glass door at one side, as the focal point. I step out of the door which has a roof overhang, and this is where people stand and smoke, but Dee tells me they eat out here sometimes in summer, at the chained-down picnic table.

On one side of the lounge there are wipe-clean vinyl settees and chairs and on the other side is a TV, housed in a wooden cabinet which is unmoveable and has Perspex covering the front with drilled holes to let the sound out. When I mention this to Denise she tells me there have been some incidents in the past where the TV has been thrown or broken.

Moving through to the kitchen, there is a pale wood effect dining table in front of the kitchen hatch. I have noticed that every kitchen has a hatch for serving food, which I later learn is because some clients are not allowed to enter the kitchen. To the left of this room is a computer cabinet and a member of staff appears to be working on the PC. A client (Teresa) is sitting at the empty table and she grins, very pleased to see us. I ask her if she remembers me from the Women's Action Group meetings and she makes a 'thinking' face, and then asks me if I would like to see her bedroom. I feel a little nosy, but she clearly wants to show it to me. The bedrooms are down a side corridor from the lounge, and at the end of the corridor is another full length glass door. Denise accompanies us and tells me that Teresa is a very tidy person, and her room is indeed very tidy. There are lots of items in her room, including CDs and DVDs, many colourful furnishings and cushions and large pictures on the walls that have been coloured in, Betty Boop, Tatty Teddy. The very large window is frosted glass. The room is very spacious but does not have an en-suite like some of the others have. There is a communal bathroom with a bath but no shower. I remark that the room is very tidy, and say thanks for letting me look round.

(Fieldnotes, LSU)

I found that the physical features of the flats had a considerable influence on the atmosphere. Long et al. (2011) emphasise the importance of architecture when planning mental health services for women. They highlight the need for neutral areas for therapeutic encounters, the sight of nature outside and a homely atmosphere (see also von Sommaruga Howard, 2004). To maximise the benefit of the built environment, they suggest close collaboration among architects, clinicians and patients at the planning stage. Although I do not know whether this was the case at Unit C, there was much visible nature outside, and large windows on the LSU providing plenty of natural light. However, the internal architecture seemed to have been designed for surveillance throughout, so there were no private areas and no neutral spaces for therapeutic encounters other than bedrooms. The manager told me that she was aware of this and was working towards creating another room at the request of clients. The lack of neutral spaces for discussion and privacy was an important issue which I will return to a number of times throughout this work.

Being shown around was helpful in getting to know people; although the wards were new to me, it did not take long for me to be included in conversations. I was curious to find more out about the people who lived and worked on the unit.

Women

Spending more time with the women, I began to find out why they were there, and how they felt when they first arrived. Most of them were welcoming and friendly and we built up relationships during my time on the wards. A good example of this is my relationship with Annie.

Asking Annie for consent to be interviewed

I sit in the lounge with Annie as she has come out of her room. I ask her why she didn't attend the community meeting, and she says, 'Because it's a load of shit.' She also tells me she's going to stop going to the WAG (women's group) because that's also shit. I say it would be good if she carried on because she is a big part of the group. She refuses. Tanya comes to sit with us. Staff members come in and go out and talk about what is happening in the other flats, but they don't mention any details or names. The TV is on and it is audible this time but there are many interruptions so nobody is really watching it. Tanya says she has a meeting about her discharge and I ask her if she will be interviewed for my study before she goes. She agrees and gives me a big smile. I ask Annie if she will be interviewed and she says simply 'no'. I ask her if I can ask her again about this another time and she just says 'no'.

(Fieldnotes, LSU)

A second meeting with Annie

After gaining enthusiastic consent to interview Annie a few days later when she approached me, I ask her what she does in the evenings. She tells me that she enjoys doing her jigsaws; she is holding a Toy Story one. I ask if she watches TV and she said that they were told by a male member of staff that they weren't allowed to watch 'One Born Every Minute'. Tanya comments that, 'Giving birth is a natural part of life.' Then Annie tells me that a member of staff was winding her up on Friday night by not letting them watch 'Embarrassing Bodies'. He said it was 'inappropriate'. The female staff member tells her that he might have been embarrassed, and I ask what the rules are with films. Annie tells me they're not allowed to watch 18 rated films and I remark that some 18 films have horrible things in. Annie says, 'We are adults you know.' I think about how to reply. I say, 'I know that, but some 18 films I would be very scared watching.' Annie says, 'You're just sticking up for him because he is a staff.' She looks angry and tells the staff that she is feeling anxious because she is remembering something that happened the other night. She turns away from me.

I try to talk to Annie after this but she doesn't want to talk to me. When I ask her a question she takes a while to answer and doesn't seem as happy to talk. I feel rebuffed.

(Fieldnotes, LSU)

Writing a letter with Annie

This is the first time I visit the flat after obtaining consent from most people. When I enter reception, I tell them that I want to see Annie. [Staff member] says 'Do you mind me asking what about? Only, she's not been very happy recently.' I tell her that Annie volunteered to write a letter at the WAG and I'm going to see if she wants any help. [Staff member] says 'Oh that's OK, she loves anything to do with the WAG, she's very enthusiastic about it.'

When I walk into the lounge of the flat, there is Annie, a male staff member and two clients. They are all sitting in the lounge, watching TV. The TV is barely audible and Annie talks to the male staff member in a loud voice as do all the staff who walk through the lounge. On the TV is some sort of Technicolor film from the 50s about Roman Centurions. When I ask all present what they are watching, they say 'Something to do with Romans.' Nobody seems interested in the program, it is interrupted constantly by people coming through and talking, but the clients have nothing else to do but to watch; it seems a comforting distraction today. I ask Annie if she wants to do the letter and she seems very enthusiastic, she gives me a lovely smile which lights up her face. She leads me to her room, which has very few personal possessions in it. Sellotaped haphazardly to the wall is a large coloured-in picture of a Disney fairy and three family photos. She has some soft toys dotted about, but no CDs or books. Her pillow is at the bottom of her bed which creaks enormously when she sits on it. I sit on a vinyl-covered chair next to the bed.

Annie's clothes are masculine and shapeless, she is wearing much worn jogging trousers and a t-shirt. Her arms are deeply scarred from old cuts and she has about 30 new scratches which run the opposite way to the scars and look sore. Annie gets a box out to lean on when writing the letter. It is a Winnie the Pooh 36 piece giant floor jigsaw; it is for age 2+.

She gets out the notes from the WAG which suggest what to write in the letter. Together we compose a letter asking management for funding so the members can do the Race for Life[2] at a nearby park. Annie is quite certain about some of the sentences she is going to put in. She needs my help to spell many words, but forms her letters competently. She does not sign the letter, saying she doesn't want to get the blame for it, and writes that it is from the WAG. She tells me that she thinks her writing looks like that of a three year old, but I say that the writing is better than mine. I do not ask her anything personal because I am worried about her state of mind after what I've been told, but really she seems quite positive, apart from complaining about her creaky bed ('they have tried to fix it but they can't') and *her door which makes strange noises at night. She thanks me for helping her and we go through to the lounge.*

In the lounge again, Annie offers me a cup of tea and we go into the kitchen. She gets out plastic cups and one plastic glass. She says 'I suppose I'd better make [name of client] one' and proceeds to make a cup of tea in the plastic glass and then water it down considerably with cold water to cool it. There is a pan full of Bolognese sauce on the stove and we remark how nice it smells. I am still wary of asking too many questions. We go back into the lounge and Annie introduces me to the male member of staff, saying that everywhere he has moved to, she has followed. He proceeds to talk about his holiday coming up. Annie puts her hand on his over the arms of the chairs and he doesn't pull away. The TV is still on quietly and one client is staring at it.

Annie is gently ribbing the male staff member. Her conversation is funny and I don't feel excluded from it, she is trying to make me feel comfortable. She is bold, free-spirited and open. She has a curious combination of over-confidence and fragility which is extremely appealing. Half of me wants to mother her and half of me wants to be her friend.

(Fieldnotes, LSU)

I have used these fieldnotes to show how engaged I became with the people on Unit C. I did become friendly with many of the clients and some of them said how much they liked having me around. They talked to me about their families, their lives and relationships on the unit, and their hopes and dreams for the future, all of which were extremely important to them, as I will show. During the first few visits, I began to find out more about the women and how they had come to be at the unit.

Women who live at the unit

Despite some literature suggesting that learning disabled people may have difficulties with temporal perception, all of the women I asked knew exactly how long they had lived at the unit, with most telling me the date they arrived. The women had lived at this hospital for between 5 months and 19 years. Four out of the 16 women I interviewed had lived at the hospital for longer than 15 years. Most of the women had come here from other units or hospitals, some from private services and one came from prison. One woman told me some details about her admittance to hospital:

Bonnie: Police rang my mum up and says 'We want to section Bonnie' and she says, 'Go for it,' because she was fed up of seeing me in the papers trying to kill myself and stuff like that. So yes she had a help with it, but I don't regret it, I've had all the help I can get now and this is it now, this is my last step to community.

(Interview, client, LSU)

The unit's website describes the service users as having complex needs, and the ostensible client group involves those who have committed offences or who have been removed from other services because of their behaviour. I became aware that pathways into the service are more complex than this.

Reasons for being in the unit – 'I've got an idea of why I'm here'

Most women told me that they were in the unit because of their behaviour, mainly aggression or self-harm. One woman mentioned that she had committed an offence, another said she had been involved with drugs, and one person said she had been moved here because she was having sexual intercourse whilst living at her previous unit (see Chapter 4 for more information). Two people said they were not sure about why they were at the service, for example:

Marion: Well in a roundabout way yes, I will say I've got an idea of why I'm here. Then again, I may be wrong. I've got a rough idea of why I'm here.

(Interview, client, LSU)

Lindsay et al. (2004) analysed a cohort of offenders with learning disabilities and found that for women, assault-related offences (including alcohol-related assault) were the most common at 33%, with breach of the peace, theft and prostitution also prevalent. In the same study they found that 66% of learning disabled women in secure care may have a significant mental illness, which Williams et al. (2004:32) argue could be described as a response to, or a creative way of coping with, 'damaging experiences that are rooted in their lived experiences of inequality and abuses of power'.

Stafford (1999) carried out a survey of case-register data for all patients resident in English high security hospitals in 1997 and found that most of the women came from deprived communities, an indicator of low social class. Most had experienced early abandonment or loss of carer followed by problematic stays in foster homes, resulting in over a third ending up in Children's Homes. Over 80% of women had not experienced a stable partnership as an adult. A combination of early trauma alongside failures of community provision to meet the needs of these women resulted in incarceration in secure hospital environments. This suggests that attachment issues may be relevant for these women, but they are not being acknowledged, and I will return to this later in my work.

Hayes (2007:190) concludes that 'this sub-group will tend to be socially disadvantaged, victims of previous sexual, physical and emotional abuse, and often suffering from mental health problems.' Both learning disabled and non-learning disabled children who have been the victim of abuse exhibit aggressive and domineering behaviours, and low self-esteem – responses which some literature associates with offending behaviours (Mansell et al., 1998). It is apparent that women in this group are subjected to the combined intersectional oppressions of low social class along with gender and disability discrimination and I will explore this further in my concluding chapter.

Here, one staff member describes her ideas about the connection between early experiences, learning disabilities and incarceration:

Adele: But it's almost like a double whammy, because people honestly have had their past experiences and often traumatic and abusive and neglectful perhaps and huge problems with attachment, and a learning disability. So there's a sense in which having a learning disability maybe makes you a bit more vulnerable to not being able to cope with these really difficult experiences as well. So you perhaps have some developmental delay, and then if you have an emotionally abusive or difficult experiences on top of that as well, I think what happens is any learning disability is compounded, so you almost get a bit stuck – particularly if it's traumatic, what's happened to people – so then they, perhaps understandably, develop pretty maladaptive or difficult ways of coping. But actually what are adaptive for them at the time.

(Interview, qualified staff)

Adele suggests that the combination between difficult life experiences and learning disabilities provokes ways of coping that result in people getting 'stuck' with maladaptive ways of managing. She claims that these ways of coping may have worked at the time for that person, but now need to change; this is why clients are at Unit C.

Life experiences – 'I've had a shit life'

All of the staff made reference to the negative life experiences of the women they cared for, and as I spent more time on the unit, the women started to tell me some of their stories. Many of their stories were very difficult to listen to and stayed with me for a long time afterwards. I give a small sample of individuals' experiences here as illustrations, but I do not attach pseudonyms for ethical reasons as it could identify clients to some readers:

* *She starts to tell me about her family. Two of her brothers are in jail, another brother died at 13, which is why her mum 'went mad'. She tells me about seeing him in the coffin and the story of how he died. She says that when she was ten, just after he died, she slit her own throat and cut her wrists and her arms. At fifteen she took pills to try and kill herself. When she came round she told the nurse they should have let her die, but the nurse said she was just doing her job. Her father died when she was 3, which she says she's glad about. He used to beat her mum and once he kidnapped her sister. She remembers being strapped in her buggy just in a nappy and her father pushed the buggy outside in the snow while he was arguing with her mum. (Fieldnotes)*

- I lost twins. And when I was 20, about 3 days before my 21st birthday I got raped and injected with heroin. And then I lost my other baby, so I've lost three kids in the space of two years. And I lost control, I lost it completely and basically I've got stronger. If it wasn't for the hospitals that I've been in I'd have been dead by now. I'd have been dead. I haven't told anybody about this because I didn't want the sympathy, because both pregnancies was due to violence that I lost them, due to violence. (Interview with client)
- So I've had a shit life, been in and out of care from the age of 2, finally put in care till I was 18, that's when all the trouble started. Left on my own to fend for myself, no social services just me on my own. (Interview with client)
- No, it was just when my mum and dad died and my then, and my sister between them, three of them died in a month. Yeah three of them died in a month, I just lost it and I've been angry ever since. I am calm now, I am calmer now than what I was when I first come in here. (Interview with client)
- [My sister] was going down once a month because I was so ill, 'cos I lived in a flat and she was going down and going food shopping or Christmas shopping and I would give her my benefits and she'd go and spend some of it on me and she'd say "I'm going to take the other half home for next week", and it would never come to me, I wasn't getting it. I had about £200 in benefits a week or a month or something, and she was keeping like a hundred out of it or something like that. She was keeping half. (Interview with client)
- *She tells me about finding her mum with slashed wrists in the bath when she was 17, she tried to bandage them and ended up dragging her mum out of the bath and tying her wrists behind her back to stop her touching them. (Fieldnotes)*
- My brother poured a kettle of boiling water on me . . . [When I came here] I have nowhere to live. My sisters don't want me, my brother don't want me. I'd nothing. (Interview with client)
- Well, I was abused from 2 till I was 8. And basically, and, that's my brother, my next door neighbour, my uncle and my dad. My dad got two years, he got found guilty for two years but the others got off. But since that happened, my sister won't have nothing to do with us because she says I'm a marriage wrecker and home breaker. And then I got told that I'd got to be put into care till I was 18, whereas my two brothers and my sister stayed with my mum. I haven't lived with my mum since I was 8 years old. (Interview with client)
- I was gang raped by my dad and some of his friends. (Interview with client)

These experiences illustrate that the women have had to deal with physical and sexual abuse as children, sexual and domestic violence, traumatic bereavement, financial abuse, and feeling left with nowhere to turn. Literature shows that many women who offend have abusive and traumatic pasts and that staff may find it difficult to know how to deal with this (Warner, 1996; Warner and Wilkins, 2004; Wilkins and Warner, 2001; Williams et al., 2004). During my time on the wards, I did not witness staff talking with clients about their pasts; however, this may have been down to the constraints of time and confidentiality.

First impressions of ward

I asked all clients how they felt when they first saw the unit. Seven people reported that they were scared, mainly because of the barriers at the entrance, and level of visible security measures such as fencing. Three people said they felt nervous, and one person felt 'devastated' because she had been told she was just coming for a visit. In fact, two women reported to me that they hadn't been told that they were staying until they arrived on the ward, for example:

Lorna: It felt weird, really weird because I just walked in with my staff from my old place, and they said, 'This is where you're going to be living now Lorna.' and I said, 'I'm not, I'm going back with my staff, this is just a visit.' They were like, 'It's not, you're staying here for real.' I was like, 'I don't want to!' but I ended up staying here. And then one of the girls came up to me and shook my hand and said 'Are you alright?' And said 'Come on, sit over here with us.' And in the end the staff stayed a little bit with me from my old place, and then they had to go. But I was devastated, I was like, 'I want to come back with you.'

(Interview, client, LSU)

Lack of information and feeling kept in the dark was a very strong theme which ran throughout my research. It seems that to avoid disturbance, clients had not been informed about important changes in their lives; however, this resulted in significant distress in the long term due to the added aspect of feeling denied important information (I will discuss the control of information more in Chapter 5). Literature points to learning disabled people often being denied information due to notions of protection and paternalism (Dein and Williams, 2008; Tuffrey-Wijne et al., 2009).

Settling in

Some of the women told me that they were so distressed on admission that they were put straight into the seclusion area, setting them apart straight away. Building up relationships with other clients is an important aspect of settling in and women told me that feeling accepted by the other women on their flat was a turning point. I noticed that newer clients talked about their families and previous lives much more than those who had lived on the unit for longer. Many women connected 'settling in' with 'learning the rules'. Here, a member of staff talked about this process:

Jackie: A lot of our clients are fairly mobile, streetwise, they've survived various experiences haven't they really? So, that's what happens I think when they come here, they understandably they come in and think, 'What's this place about? What can I expect from here?' And I think what happens quite quickly is, they start to think there's various rules and things that you do and that you don't do, and they need to fit in with that. And then, perhaps as part of that process, then well, 'If I keep my head down and I do as I'm told, then I'll be okay.' But part of that process is then 'Well, if I do as the staff tell me' – you maybe lose a bit of confidence and a few skills maybe? I don't know. But then after a while, there's something about the shift is really around people's lives are orchestrated externally, so they maybe have a sense of 'Well, I don't necessarily have as much of a voice.'

(Interview, qualified staff)

Jackie pointed out that people's lives are 'orchestrated externally' and because of this clients lose some of their 'voice' and skills by abiding by the rules. This is related to Parry-Crooke et al.'s (2000) study, where service users reported that they felt rules were sometimes arbitrary and could change day-to-day, and that they had to learn the rules through experience. Interestingly, Jackie equated following the rules with passivity, a loss of confidence and skills, something that I will return to in Chapter 5.

Staff entry into the service

The staff I interviewed consisted of support workers, qualified nursing staff, managers and one clinical psychologist (who I have described as 'qualified staff' to preserve anonymity). As with clients, most of the staff also told me that they were 'afraid' or 'apprehensive' when they first started working at the service. The literature recommends that staff should be recruited specifically to work with women, (Parry-Crooke and Stafford, 2009; Sarkar and di Lustro, 2011), but this was not the case with any of my participants. However, all of the staff I had interviewed had arrived before the introduction of single-sex wards in 2002 (Department of Health, 2000) and therefore this specification may have been incorporated into current recruitment policy. Monica told me:

Monica: I was frightened to death at first, I didn't like it. I was frightened of the clients and I suppose coming is as a new person, I found the staff very cliquey, which now I think, 'Oh well we're not like that at all', but new people coming in, I bet they do find that . . . And then I got assaulted by one of the female clients, she pulled my hair, but she pulled me off a chair. I was sat in the office and she pulled me out of the office with my hair . . . It was horrible. So then I remember ringing my mum and saying, 'I can't work here, it's not what I wanted to do. I want to look after people and care for people, I don't want to do this.'

(Interview, qualified staff)

Other staff mentioned feeling nervous and wary of clients, with some staff feeling confused about how to work with a forensic population; qualified nursing staff told me that their nurse training had been directed towards physical care and treatment of people with more significant impairments. Staff mentioned being unaware of the differing experiences and needs of women when they first started work. However, progress was being made: whilst I was spending time on the unit, 'gender' training courses were beginning to be offered to staff, which covered issues such as child sexual abuse and how this can affect women's current behaviour. The activities of the WAG group added to the visibility of women in the unit and all this knowledge filtered into day-to-day life on the unit as I will show. Furthermore, female clients were involved in training staff about self-harm. There was clearly an increasing interest in the women at the unit, as further evidenced by the approval of my research proposal, so it seems that in the future staff may be more prepared and knowledgeable about the women at the service.

The service – day-to-day

The women live on single-sex flats with between two and eight people. The daily routine is similar for all women, meals are taken together, and day services sessions run at the same time each day. Each person has a day each week put aside for 'domestic skills' which means they spend the day on the ward, cleaning the flat and washing their clothes. Day services activities are individually planned and clients take activities off the wards, such as crafts, cooking and education which involves basic literacy and numeracy skills. In the evening, some clients are able to go to 'the club' where they can play pool and listen to music.

Day services – 'I think it's babyish'

Many of the clients were pleased with the variation of day services on offer, and those who came from other services in particular pointed out that they were happy with the day activities, which they called 'work'. Some of the women worked in the gardens and they enjoyed being outside. Most of the women commented, however, that some of the activities could be childish, for example:

Rebecca: What do you think about day services, your work and everything?
Marion: Basically I don't like day services, I think it's childish I think it's babyish. I think I'm more, I'm more of an adult. Well, I'm nearly [age – 40s] next month and all we're doing is go to work and draw pictures and colour them in but for me, I'm more grown up, I'm more intelligent than most people are. Not that I'm calling anybody or slagging them down, the patients. I'm more mature and I like to do things to my standard, I just don't basically like going.

(Interview, client, LSU)

A number of clients pointed out the futility of colouring in. I did accompany clients to day services and saw some of this happening; colouring in, making boxes and small craft items. Staff members were also concerned about the activities being very basic and not offering life skills, for example:

John: And the people working [in day services] aren't teachers, they're support workers. There used to be a farm and cement works, upholstery. They still do a lot now, they make bean bags and the print shop's good. They make all the books that we have and things like that. A lot of people say it's repetitive but it focuses them. Some of the clients absolutely love it, [client] loves print-shop, she's making books, she feels like she's doing something. The allotments is good but arts and crafts – I think some of the clients are treated like children to be honest.

(Interview, unqualified staff)

John talked about work in the institution when it was housing non-forensic people, who were working (unpaid) for the upkeep of the institution. Since the move to community-based provision, this type of work has been rejected in policy for obvious reasons, although the replacements offered seemed to disregard any sort of skills which may be useful in the community. John went on to say that he thought day services should be more skills-based, preparing people for when they move back to the community:

John: Personally I've said it for years, you know the [nearby shop]? I thought [Unit C] should have bought that and all clients then had to buy their cigarettes and toiletries from there, and clients could run it. A lot of the skills they're learning here, they're not going to use. A lot of clients if you asked them how much a loaf of bread were they wouldn't have a clue, they just know how much a vending machine is. It's just life skills really, basic.

(Interview, unqualified staff)

Like John, some staff were concerned about the lack of life skills being taught. When asked how day services could be improved, both staff and clients suggested work which was more useful and off-site, such as swimming and cycling, looking after animals, voluntary work placements helping other people and taking mainstream college courses such as learning sign language.

Day services were mandatory, referred to as 'work' – and there were implications for those who did not attend as I will show in Chapter 6. According to Goffman (1961), a marked difference between institutional life and that of ordinary society is that of work: 'There will be different motives for work and different attitudes towards it. This is a basic adjustment required of the inmates and those who must induce them to work' (Goffman, 1961:20). Further, McWade (2014:107) shows how the inability to work is equated with sickness in late capitalist societies; therefore work is considered to restore a person's 'normative subject position'. McWade shows the assumed value of work in concepts of rehabilitation of psychiatric patients, and how this reduces creativity. Along with McWade, I would agree that creative pursuits such as art and music-making may be more advantageous to clients' self-esteem. As Carlson puts it:

Through forms of artistic expression, the very meaning of the 'good life' may be reimagined, thereby leaving behind models of disability that are restricted to pathology, normalization, function, and cure.

(Carlson, 2013:99)

Encouragingly, as I completed my fieldwork, the Unit were employing occupational therapy practitioners to overhaul the day services system. This was expected to bring about a huge improvement in day services provision, as one of the qualified staff members pointed out:

Karen: It'll take time to bed down like everything but it'll be fabulous.
Rebecca: So what will their role be, organising a programme for each client?
Karen: But individually based, person-centred to their needs. Which is massive, it's really important and it'll work in relation to their treatment and care plans so it will all be together; it will be miles better.

(Interview, qualified staff)

Karen was very enthusiastic about this new development and had high expectations. Person-centred day services seem like a good idea, but it was evident that the selection and type of activities needs to be improved also. Utilising community activities for those who are allowed, would be a step forward. One encouraging provision for women was the WAG group, where women and their staff would meet and discuss issues of relevance to them. Women would join for six months at a time, and would each take on a role at the meeting, for example chair, minutes, tea and coffee etc. Events would also be organised for the WAG, such as charity coffee mornings and cake bakes, and organising a group of women to join the charity fun-run in the community. Women really enjoyed making a contribution to this group, as I showed earlier with Annie's letter writing.

Evening/social activities – 'I like washing pots up'

Evening activities varied depending on which area of the service (low or medium secure) women lived in. Most women talked about watching TV, and spending time in their room if they were able. All of the women went to buy drinks, sweets or crisps from the vending machine (vendor) in an evening. Here, Bella describes her evening activities on the medium secure ward.

Bella: I go to me room roughly about quarter past six, I watch Hollyoaks and The Simpsons and then I do some writing from half six until seven, then I watch Eastenders and then at half seven I come out and to the vendor, I sit around with me bottle of drink or me crisps or whatever I get. Then at about eight o'clock, sometimes I sit out all night with the girls, depending on who's on [staff members], or sometimes I go back to me room and read or have a little sleep or tidying up me room. Always busy, I'm always busy I'm never still . . . At any time we can do board games, I've got jigsaw puzzles anyway, so I can do jigsaw puzzles. I've got me own art and crafts stuff, so I can do art and stuff, I can't have scissors, but I can use supervised scissors. I can be supervised using a pencil sharpener, so I can do all that of a night-time, the staff don't mind doing that. Obviously I can't write if clients are causing problems.

(Interview, client, MSU)

Despite Bella seeming very happy with the evening activities, Helen was less so. She would have liked to go to the club on the MSU; however, there was only one club for both men and women, and women were limited in their access to this social space due to staffing:

Helen: We just watch TV really and go to the vendor, and then we just have supper, watch TV and go to bed.
Rebecca: What would you like to do?
Helen: I'd like to have chance to mix with people but there's not enough staff.
(Interview, client, MSU)

On the LSU, similar evening activities were described:

Rebecca: What kind of things do you do in the evenings?
Marion: I like watching TV, I like writing letters, I like reading and all that. And just talking to my friends and another thing I like doing is, I like washing pots up and putting them all away.
(Interview, client, LSU)

From what the clients were saying, evening social activities were quite limited. The Unit had organised a 'woman's hour' when LSU women were able to go into the grounds and meet for 45 minutes in a specific area, although some women found it difficult to access due to needing staff to go with them. This resulted in many women residing on the wards in the evenings. Here a member of staff pointed out that when designing and building the new MSU building, women's evening activities were not considered to be a priority:

Adele: Women are obviously in the minority in the service, so if we start back at the beginning, one of the things when we were building the MSU was they very definitely separated off the women's flat, the women's garden, the women shouldn't be out on the corridor in their pyjamas when the men were out in the corridor in their pyjamas getting their medication and so they've got a separate medication room and all the rest of it. I can clearly remember before the building was finished, being shown round it and I asked very pointedly, 'So if that's the social space, where's the women's social space?', 'Well they're in with the men.' I said, 'But they're separated for everything else, they've even got their own garden and yet you're expecting them just to socialise with the men?' So there was that, there was some not recognising that they may actually want separate social space; they may not, but there was no facility being built in in case they did. There are times in the social space where it's females only, but that took a bit of doing, that wasn't there in the first year that we opened it up. So there's things like that where there still feels to be a bit of a struggle to actually recognise that women may want to have a separate space and may not always want to be in with the men. I remember it took ages to get pampering sessions and female-only sessions recognised in the works and the social bit and all the rest. So it still feels like a bit of an uphill struggle sometimes.

(Interview, qualified staff)

Adele described how difficult it was to design a medium secure unit with women in mind, pointing out that women may want a separate social space. Much of the discussion around women and their activities included mentions of 'pampering' sessions. Many of the staff, when asked about facilities that they would like to see for women talked about provision for hair and beauty sessions. They wanted staff to be allowed to provide these sessions in a specific space and also for women to be taught how to groom themselves. Concern was raised in interviews about the way women look and that they may deliberately avoid personal care and grooming due to lack of awareness or as a result of their abusive pasts, for example:

Monica: I think some it's a lack of ability, that they've never known how to groom themselves and they've never had an interest, or maybe even the money to buy decent clothes. And then I think with some it's about previous abuse, that if they make themselves very unattractive people won't want to sexually abuse them. Some of them won't wash their hair or care for themselves when they're on their period because I think they think it keeps them safe and it keeps people away from them.

(Interview, qualified staff)

This example of women's past abuse being used to explain their lack of grooming was very interesting to me. It seems that, unlike much of the literature looking at histories of institutions, where women were discouraged from thinking about their appearance (Atkinson et al., 2000; Barron, 2002) or, as described in Chapter 2, research which showed women's attire as highly regulated (Phillips, 2007), grooming is perceived and handled in a more nuanced way at Unit C, with staff acknowledging contextual and experiential reasons for women's choices. However, most women did seem to enjoy the 'pamper sessions' when they went ahead, and found them relaxing. Some enjoyed the women only spaces and activities at Unit C, although would have liked more variety of activities. With the exception of two women, the women I spoke to also valued the opportunity to spend time with men, either at work during the day or in the evenings at the club; for example when I asked about a new policy where women and men were being separated in the evenings, Katrina explained:

Katrina: [It feels like] Crap. Seeing my boyfriend was the only reason I went to the club at night. [I feel] segregated.

(Interview, client, LSU)

Although most women wanted to spend time with men, saying that it reflected 'normal life', there were women who did not, evidencing the need for separate social and working spaces.

Security – 'A proper locked up place'

My fieldwork focussed on two wards on the LSU, and one ward in the MSU. The level of security was much more noticeable in the medium secure unit, as the following fieldnotes illustrate:

> The MSU building is surrounded by a two-storey fence. To enter the MSU, you need to enter the large double height lobby. Then you must be let into the 'bubble' where doors are locked in front of you and behind, and hand over your 'key card'. In return you get a pouch with a belt for around your waist, a bunch of keys on a length of webbing and a fob which allows you to pass through shared doors without using a key. You also get a 'blick' which has a panic button and would sound an alarm when pulled off your belt, the blick sounds alarms every so often when a member of staff has raised the alarm, and has a display which tells you which room to go to if you are able to respond. You need to thread all of these onto the belt before you can pass out of the 'bubble.' You also must sign a form to say you do not have any of the contraband items, such as a phone or cigarette lighter. Every door is locked, even bedroom and bathroom doors. The seclusion room hatch, about a foot wide and at waist height, is unlocked by using two separate keys at the same time.
>
> (Fieldnotes)

The level of security is maintained both on the MSU and LSU by locked doors. All entrance and kitchen doors are locked on the LSU and alarms sound if they stay unlocked for more than a few seconds. On the MSU, people rarely leave the building as all-day services are on site. Service users from the LSU attend work which is situated in different buildings from where they live; they are escorted in small groups or 'one-to-one' by staff members to work and picked up afterwards.

This level of security is often distressing for the women, as Kate pointed out when remembering how she felt when she first arrived:

Kate: I felt very scared, especially when I got to the gates and realised they were locked gates because they were then, and em, you know security, I thought, 'Woah, this is more like a proper locked up place.'

(Interview, client, LSU)

The women seemed to equate the level of security with a penal regime when they first arrived. Even though Teresa had mainly positive things to say about the low secure unit, she particularly did not like the security:

Teresa: [I'd like them to] Unlock the doors. That's why I call it a 24/7 because they are locking the doors now. That main door out there will be locked.
Rebecca: Does that bother you?

Teresa:	Yes.
Rebecca:	Why?
Teresa:	Other flats, people who are there runs away.
Rebecca:	And that's why they lock the door? How does that make you feel?
Teresa:	It's like prison, it is and that's why I'm saying! It's 24/7.

(Interview, client, LSU)

Teresa felt as though she was being punished with locked doors because of the risk of other people absconding. She considered this to be unfair as she was not at risk of running away. Staff members likewise talked about physical security as less necessary to the women than encouraging feelings of safety through relationships, for example:

Karen: These women are so vulnerable and so damaged that they need to feel safe. And the only way we can make them feel safe is to show them that we care about them by putting the boundaries in and making sure that they don't come to any harm. And they see the boundaries that we put in place as us keeping them safe.

(Interview, Staff member, MSU, qualified)

Karen's concepts of 'boundaries' refers to relational security as described in Chapter 1. Rather than physical security, such as locked doors and boundary fences, many qualified staff talked about relational security as being more important for women. Relational security relies on the staff/client relationship and is represented by high staff-client ratios, provision for staff and clients to spend time together, providing a balance between openness and intrusion, and high levels of trust (Parry-Crooke and Stafford, 2009).

Conclusion

This work allowed me the privileged position of hearing people talk about their lives and families, their past and current experiences and relationships. These first impressions illustrate how women, who have been exposed to gendering and disabling experiences throughout their lives, continue to be subjugated via certain practices and conventions after their arrival on Unit C. Arguably, it is their experiences of deprivation, abandonment and abuse, accompanied by the lack of support offered by community services which have contributed to their admittance to the unit. Surely, the reasoning behind their confinement in an NHS secure service rather than a prison should be to address and reconcile these issues.

Spending time on the wards enabled me to feel in part how it is to be locked in a ward, unable to exit without summoning a staff member, and this made me feel anxious even as a researcher. I found that some experiences and opinions were shared between staff and clients on Unit C; for example both staff and clients reported feeling nervous when first arriving on the unit, due to the level of visible security such as locked doors and/or expectations about the client group. One key difference between staff and clients about arriving on the unit, however, was information. Clients were not often told that they would be staying, reflecting the paternalism of services when it comes to learning disabled people. Johnson's (1998) concept of the 'mutual gaze' was also evident to me at this stage, for example when Annie was complaining about the male member of staff – there was evidence of two-way appraisal between staff and clients.

Both staff and clients were concerned about the childishness of daytime activities. Learning disability services have a history of treating people like children (Atkinson et al., 2000; Baron et al., 1999), and I was told a number of times by different women, 'We are not children', yet I was aware that there was a discourse in the service about people being 'stuck' at a certain age. Although this may reflect past experiences and show that staff are taking these into account, I do not believe this discourse to be a helpful way to talk about people. It would seem that the legacy of institutional discourses about learning disabled people is still evident. When I asked them what they would like to do, many of the women were drawn to caring activities, such as looking after animals or disabled people, evidencing the need for individualised day services. Whilst it may be impossible for some women who have committed offences to work with people, spending time with animals is a realistic expectation.

Discourse about gender, disability and social class ran throughout these first impressions, with women being appraised as lacking in ability to groom themselves or purposely neglecting their appearance. The premium placed on personal grooming for women was evident through the provision of 'pamper' sessions. These did seem to be successful, with women reporting that they enjoy them although the reasons for this may go beyond learning about beauty. Literature about attachment difficulties explains the benefits of safe, comforting touch (Heller & LaPierre, 2012). Additionally, I noticed that the perceived social class of clients was played out in the designated 'treats' and privileges, most notably visits to the 'vendor' and the choice of trips further afield. Conceptions of gender featured in notions of 'relational security', the use of the staff/client relationship to help women feel safe that was talked about as an aspect of femininity. This was in contrast to the physical security, a masculine requirement, which was manifested in the controlled environment and behaviour management techniques. Indeed, relational issues were very important to clients and staff, and I shall turn to these in the following chapter.

Notes

1 Groups of flats are referred to as 'wards' on the unit, as in hospitals. This, I think, reflects the medical intentions of the service, as an organisation that is there to 'treat' people.
2 A fundraising 5-km community run organised by Cancer Research UK each year.

Bibliography

Atkinson, D., McCarthy, M., Walmsley, J., Cooper, M., Rolph, S., Aspis, S. . . . Ferris, G. (2000). *Good times, bad times: Women with learning difficulties telling their stories.* Kidderminster: BILD Publications.

Baron, S., Riddell, S., & Wilson, A. (1999). The secret of eternal youth: Identity, risk and learning difficulties. *British Journal of Sociology of Education*, 20(4), 483–499.

Barron, K. (2002). Who am I? Women with learning difficulties (re) constructing their self-identity. *Scandinavian Journal of Disability Research*, 4(1), 58–79.

Carlson, L. (2013). Musical becoming: Intellectual disability and the transformative power of music. In M. Wappett & K. Arndt (Eds.), *Foundations of disability studies* (pp. 83–104). New York: Palgrave Macmillan.

Dein, K., & Williams, P. (2008). Relationships between residents in secure psychiatric units: Are safety and sensitivity really incompatible? *Psychiatric Bulletin*, 32(8), 284.

Department of Health. (2000). *Secure futures for women*. London: Department of Health.

Goffman, E. (1961). *Asylums: Essays on the social situation of mental patients and other inmates*. New York: Anchor Books, Doubleday & Co.

Hayes, S. (2007). Women with learning disabilities who offend: What do we know? *British Journal of Learning Disabilities*, 35(3), 187–191.

Heller, L., & LaPierre, A. (2012). *Healing developmental trauma*. Berkeley: North Atlantic Books.

Johnson, K. (1998). *Deinstitutionalising women: an ethnographic study of institutional closure*. Cambridge, UK: Cambridge Univ Press.

Lindsay, W., Smith, A., Quinn, K., Anderson, A., Smith, A., Allan, R., & Law, J. (2004). Women with intellectual disability who have offended: Characteristics and outcome. *Journal of Intellectual Disability Research*, 48(6), 580–590.

Long, C. G., Langford, V., Clay, R., Craig, L., & Hollin, C. R. (2011). Architectural change and the effects on the perceptions of the ward environment in a medium secure unit for women. *The British Journal of Forensic Practice*, 13(3), 205–212.

Mansell, S., Sobsey, D., & Moskal, R. (1998). Clinical findings among sexually abused children with and without developmental disabilities. *Mental Retardation*, 36, 12–22.

Mcwade, B. (2014). *Recovery in an "arts for mental health" unit*. Ph.D. Thesis, Lancaster University.

Parry-Crooke, G., Oliver, C., & Newton, J. (2000). *Good girls: Surviving the secure system, a consultation with women in high and medium secure psychiatric settings*. London: Women in Special Hospitals (WISH).

Parry-Crooke, G., & Stafford, P. (2009). *My life: In safe hands?* London: Metropolitan University.

Phillips, D. (2007). Embodied narratives: Control, regulation and bodily resistance in the life course of older women with learning difficulties. *European Review of History – Revue européenne d'Histoire*, 14(4), 503–524.

Sarkar, J., & di Lustro, M. (2011). Evolution of secure services for women in England. *Advances in Psychiatric Treatment*, 17(5), 323–331.

Scior, K. (2003). Using discourse analysis to study the experiences of women with learning disabilities. *Disability & Society*, 18(6), 779–795.

Stafford, P. (1999). *Defining gender issues: Redefining women's services*. London: Women in Secure Hospitals (WISH).

Tuffrey-Wijne, I., Bernal, J., Hubert, J., Butler, G., & Hollins, S. (2009). People with learning disabilities who have cancer: An ethnographic study. *British Journal of General Practice*, 59(564), 503–509.

von Sommaruga Howard, T. (2004). The physical environment and use of space. In P. Campling, S. Davies & G. Farquharson (Eds.), *From toxic institutions to therapeutic environments: Residential settings in mental health services* (pp. 69–78). New York: Springer.

Warner, S. (1996). *Visibly special? Women, child sexual abuse and special hospitals.* Aldershot: Avebury.

Warner, S., & Wilkins, T. (2004). Between subjugation and survival: Women, borderline personality disorder and high security mental hospitals. *Journal of Contemporary Psychotherapy*, 34(3), 265–278.

Wilkins, T., & Warner, S. (2001). Women in special hospitals: Understanding the presenting behaviour of women diagnosed with borderline personality disorder. *Journal of Psychiatric and Mental Health Nursing*, 8(4), 289–297.

Williams, J., Scott, S., & Bressingham, C. (2004). Dangerous journeys: Women's pathways into and through secure mental health services. In N. Jeffcote & T. Watson (Eds.), *Working therapeutically with women in secure mental health settings: Forensic focus 27* (pp. 31–43). London: Jessica Kingsley Publishers.

4   Relationships on the locked ward

The largest section of my analysis for this study concerned relationships. Learning disabled women have been described as basing their 'sense of self' (Becker, 1997:98) on the relational experiences throughout their lives (see also Atkinson et al., 2000; Sarkar and di Lustro, 2011). Relationships on Unit C, however, were seen to be inherently problematic for learning disabled women, as evidenced by staff comments about clients' past relationships and their effect on current relationships, such as the following:

Rebecca: Why do you think women are considered to be so difficult to deal with?

Adele: I think a big part of it is down to their experience of disruptive relationships in childhood definitely, some of it is down to learning disability, obviously in terms of the cognitive ability to understand what relationships are all about and how to go about it. Somebody with a learning disability for example, one of their features may be impulsive behaviour and not understanding social norms of keeping a polite space from people and invading people's space and stuff like that, because that applies to a lot of people with learning disability, not just people who've had problems in the past. So you often get a situation where just because somebody has reciprocated a 'hello' at the club the person takes it for granted that they're now their girlfriend or their boyfriend. It's about teaching people, in therapy or by role modelling behaviour on the ward, teaching people what a normal reciprocal relationship is, what a friendship is, how you start off with a hierarchy of friendship if you like. That you've got your colleagues and they become friends and then they become closer friends and then they become intimate friends, but a lot of people with learning disability want to jump from associate to intimate friend without going through the stages of getting to know somebody. For a lot of people that's what they're in here to learn as much as anything else, the norms of expectation.

(Interview, qualified staff)

Adele very clearly pointed out that a feature of learning disability (in her opinion) is the difficulty to establish proper and correct relationships. However, she did suggest that people can learn the norms of friendship and intimate relationships, and that a principal role of the service was to teach this to people. A Disability Studies perspective would take into account the lack of opportunities offered for learning disabled people to establish relationships throughout their lives, and as Adele shows, the 'norms of expectation' are always present. The literature shows how important it is for learning disabled people to be able to build supportive relationships in the community, to help them access services and to protect themselves from violence (Hollomotz, 2013). Often the things which happen to learning disabled people, such as frequent placement moves and lack of carer support, undermine their experience of building and maintaining relationships (Murphy et al., 1996). Additionally, people with abusive pasts have often experienced isolation and undermining of any supportive relationships (enforced by the abuser), and segregation in secure settings can perpetuate this isolation (Lindsay et al., 2010). Adele suggested that building relationships is an important skill; however, the way secure services work can mean that clients are frequently relocated, and continually reliant on others to tell them what to do, which traps them into the role of dependant and can undermine these abilities (McCorkell, 2011).

Borderline personality disorder and relationships

As I mentioned in my introductory chapter, some of the client participants had been diagnosed with Borderline Personality Disorder (BPD), which is a controversial diagnosis as a disorder of the personality has been traditionally described as untreatable. This is something which has changed within policy, as a staff member pointed out here:

Dawn: Historically, they've said that they're untreatable which is why it's so difficult to work with them because there's no medication that will make them, there's no medication that will make them any different . . . They're not untreatable any more! NICE [National Institute for Clinical Excellence] went absolutely nuts and a few years ago released a paper called 'No longer a diagnosis of exclusion'[1] and basically it used to be that people, I don't know about here but certainly other places, psychiatric units and stuff it was 'They've got personality disorder, ship them out because we can't treat them, there's nothing we can do about them.' And people were ignored.

(Interview, qualified staff)

Literature states that between 60% and 100% of women with this diagnosis have experienced childhood sexual abuse (Ogata et al., 1990; Stafford, 1999). Indeed, in Wilkins and Warner's analysis of the case files of 16 women diagnosed with BPD, all 16 women had experienced some form of emotional abuse during childhood, including lack of recognition of emotional needs, rejecting parenting, witnessing violence in the family, threats towards the life of the child, neglect and unstable relationships. All of the women had reported sexual abuse from someone within their immediate family, 11 reported physical abuse, seven reported severe neglect, 11 had been taken into care, 15 reported difficult relationships with their natural mother, and all reported that their communications of distress as a child were ignored (Wilkins and Warner, 2001). It is interesting in light of their past experiences, that women are given the BPD label rather than being diagnosed as having developed Post Traumatic Stress Disorder (PTSD) or an attachment disorder.

A staff member showed how BPD diagnosed women on Unit C were described as 'jealous', 'manipulative', and 'team splitting':

Dawn: They can't deal with other people having input so they want, they want the attention. They want the attention all of the time . . . the majority of people with borderline personality disorder are jealous to the utmost degree because it has to be, everything in their life is about them and everything that goes on is about them . . . [They are] masters, absolute masters at manipulating staff teams and also [they] manage to split staff teams.

(Interview, qualified staff)

Below is an example of another qualified staff member accusing women clients of 'splitting teams':

Karen: They're brilliant at it, they're brilliant. They're experts at being able to split a team, they're experts at getting something that they shouldn't have because that's all they've got to think about but it is it's part of them, part of their personality disorder.

(Interview, qualified staff)

These two examples show how these women are described in contradictory terms, as learning disabled, which in itself suggests social inability, incapable of conducting relationships as noted by Adele earlier, yet being described as 'brilliant' and 'masters' at manipulation and causing discord between staff. Iona summed this up well with:

Iona: [It was] very frustrating for the people who were embroiled in it. You could see her putting everything in a big pot and stirring them up.

(Interview, qualified staff)

Some survey studies have looked at staff perceptions of working with women with mental health conditions who were diagnosed with BPD (Markham, 2003; Markham and Trower, 2003). The staff surveyed were described as having negative opinions of those diagnosed with BPD, due to the perception that they had more ability to control their behaviour than other patients.

The attitudes of staff are critical; indeed Wilkins and Warner emphasise that therapeutic change in women diagnosed with BPD can only come about when patterns and responses are changed and re-enactments of past experiences no longer happen, in other words when women are no longer silenced or disbelieved about their experiences and are able to discuss them in a supportive environment. They suggest that raising awareness of the centrality of the trauma in women's adaptive behaviour should help staff to challenge their beliefs: 'Having a knowledge base in which to make sense of re-enactments thus serves to engender confidence and reduce defensive behaviour' (Wilkins and Warner, 2001:295). Viewing women's behaviour in light of its context is also recommended by Herman (1997), who proposes that understanding the role of childhood trauma in the development of BPD should inform every aspect of treatment:

> This understanding provides the basis for a cooperative therapeutic alliance that normalizes and validates the survivor's emotional reactions to past events, while recognizing that these reactions may be maladaptive in the present. Moreover, a shared understanding of the survivor's characteristic disturbances of relationship and the consequent risk of repeated victimization offers the best insurance against unwitting re-enactments of the original trauma in the therapeutic relationship.
>
> (Herman, 1997:127)

Literature about BPD therefore advocates the consideration of past and current experiences and how these are at risk of being repeated, hence moving away from a medicalised model and taking on a more social model approach. One staff member told me about her concept of how to treat someone diagnosed with a personality disorder:

Dawn: The only way that you can treat someone with personality disorder is through therapeutic relationships and through the different types of therapy like, DBT [Dialectical Behaviour Therapy] that we've started running here, which is about making them recognise their emotions and stuff.

(Interview, qualified staff)

Dawn's comment emphasises the role of positive and productive staff/client relationships in working with someone with personality disorder. As I was completing my research, Unit C had begun introducing Dialectical Behaviour Therapy (Linehan, 1993), by adapting this therapeutic method for learning disabled people and training therapists and staff in its use (Thomson and Johnson, 2017). Therapeutic relationships with high levels of trust and openness are endorsed in the literature as crucial to any sort of therapeutic progression for women diagnosed with personality disorder (Parry-Crooke and Stafford, 2009; Sarkar and di Lustro, 2011). DBT privileges the therapeutic relationship and teaches skills for effective relationships.

Crawford's work with learning disabled women argues that the BPD diagnosis is extremely damaging. She proposes that these diagnoses 'form the institutional perceptions of women as a group of "disorderly women", using women's distress and behaviour as evidence of further madness; and perpetuating the institutional mythology of "difficult" women' (Crawford, 2001:5). She further claims that the Borderline Personality diagnosis renders women as categorised on the edge of diagnosis, intelligence and womanhood; and she asks whether experiences of abuse or trauma can be quantified into this single diagnostic category.

My current study supports Crawford's claims. The BPD diagnosis on Unit C necessarily indicated difficulties with relationships which were considered to be individual to the woman who is diagnosed. These difficulties were described in terms of manipulative and attention-seeking behaviour, which was attributed to the individual woman rather than taking into account the context. This is a theme which recurs throughout this book.

Staff/client relationships – 'She's always been there for me'

Relationships between staff and clients are extremely important in inpatient services, indeed all therapeutic experiences are based around these, with clients reporting that relationships with staff are more important to them than therapeutic interventions *per se* (Molvaer et al., 1992; Clarkson et al., 2009). Staff have reported that engaging with and spending time with the person is important to the maintenance of their relationships with clients (Shattell et al., 2007), and staff and clients explain that trust, respect and feeling comfortable together are fundamental in this respect (Hostick and McClelland, 2002). According to the clients in Forchuk's (1998) study, trust, availability, and consistency of staff facilitated the progression of the staff/client relationship when moving through services and into the community.

On Unit C, particularly in the LSU, clients spend much of their time with staff who are often not qualified and who have many jobs to do, such as cooking, observations and paperwork. Despite these demands on staff time, I saw many types of relationship being played out on the ward. There were many examples of positive interactions between staff and clients. A good example is an exchange I saw during the Christmas celebrations:

> A couple of hours before the Christmas party is due to start, Lorna asks Candice (staff member) if she would put her some make up on. Candice brings the pallet and asks Lorna which colours she likes and gently and tenderly applies the make up to her face. Lorna is asking questions the whole time about what the party will be like and Candice is replying patiently. Lorna asks what she should do if she starts to feel anxious. Candice says that at any time she can whisper to her and she will bring her back to the ward.
>
> (Fieldnotes, MSU)

This caring interaction, which is an example of comforting touch, shows that staff can and do put much effort into the therapeutic relationship. Of course, the fact that Candice can reassure Lorna to this extent is dependent on staffing levels being sufficient enough for Candice to be able to bring Lorna back to the ward, and if this did not happen after Candice had agreed, Lorna would have felt let down. I think that the fear that this might happen is the reason why some staff appear avoidant in some of their interactions, such as:

> Annie requests to help with the weekly shop, as does Teresa when I'm there, but the staff member says 'We'll have to ask about that.' Andie joins in and asks the staff member about her birthday trip out the following week. The staff member avoids making eye contact and keeps replying that no decision has been made about it yet, she eventually says that they will discuss it another time. I think that she is wary of making promises she cannot necessarily keep.
>
> (Fieldnotes, LSU)

When I asked clients what they considered the staff's role to be, all clients replied that staff are there to help them. Responses included words such as helping, caring, listening and supporting people to move forward. Some staff also discussed how they saw their role:

John: To support them, daily needs, try and stop them from getting down and things like that. Um (pause), really it's to be a friend. A lot of it is, you know like, to be a friend to them, and be there if they need to talk, reassure them sometimes, and again if they have a bad day, they have a bad day. Everybody has a bad day, you know, it's how you react and recover.

(Interview, staff LSU)

I find it interesting that a male staff used the word 'friend' to describe the staff/client relationship, and talked about 'reassuring' and 'being there'. This emphasises the opportunities for a caring relationship to emerge, as described in the feminist literature on caring (Walmsley, 1993), which can be based on reciprocity and interdependence (Kittay, 2001; Williams and Robinson, 2001). As in the previous chapter, I saw evidence of many positive relationships between male staff and female clients. Here, a ward manager discusses the attributes that are important for staff members in building good relationships:

Karen: It's having that empathy a bit, that dividing line between empathy and 'Right, listen, we've got structure, we've got boundaries. You need to do that.' But it's having that fairness being able to say, 'No you're not going, you're not going to the vendor because . . .' And then going back to them twenty minutes later and saying, 'Are you alright, you understand why you couldn't go out?' That kind of stuff, but it's being able to do that.

(Interview, qualified staff)

Karen described the attributes that are important in direct care staff. She mentioned the balance between fairness and empathy, being able to tell somebody that they are not allowed to do something, but to also be able to understand if they are unhappy about this.

Some clients specifically discussed staff when asked about their experience of living at the unit, for example Bonnie:

Rebecca: How do you feel about living here?

Bonnie: Brilliant, I love it. We have staff that'll play cards and Connect 4 and play games with us and stuff like that. Yes, they just mingle in with us. There's staff that just sit there, there's not many staff that do sit down and do nothing, but there's staff that are really good. Especially if you're bored.

(Interview, client, LSU)

Bonnie felt that time spent with staff was very important for her. She liked playing games with staff and talked about some staff making the time to spend with clients despite having other jobs that needed doing. Kate pointed out that staff will make time for clients in certain situations such as at times of distress, unless they are doing something very important:

Rebecca: Can you think about the staff that you work with? What are the good things about the staff?

Kate: They're very helpful, like if we say 'Can we speak to you, we want to have a word with you because we're upset,' or something. They'll stop what they're doing, unless it's something like putting the sharps away. If they're putting the sharps away in the cupboard they'll say 'Just give me a minute I'm putting the sharps away' – they can't leave them around. But if it's nothing that's as serious as dropping them to talk to us, like if they were doing notes on the computer they would stop doing the notes and come and talk to us. The only time they don't do that is when they might be leaving potentially dangerous stuff around.

(Interview, client, LSU)

Kate pointed out that staff might be putting 'sharps' (knives) away in the kitchen. This is an important task and involves concentration to count the knives and complete the record form. Kate clearly indicated that availability of staff to talk to her was important.

Marion told me why she likes some of her staff, who she picked out by name:

Marion: [I like] their personalities and the way they laugh and joke with you. The way they help me, they go out of their way to help me. And like I say (name) one of the staff, have you heard of her? And (name) they're two of my favourites on here.

Rebecca: How do they help you?

Marion: Well they help me by doing my hair for me, putting my make up on when I go out places, getting my clothes ready and you know, when I'm down and all that, when I need a shoulder to cry on, them two are round when I need their help.

(Interview, client, LSU)

Marion picked out the two key aspects that clients discussed when talking about their relationships with staff, practical help and emotional support. These two key roles were highlighted as important by clients in Clarkson's (2009) paper drawing on interviews and focus groups. Annie also pointed out that practical support featured in her relationship with a staff member, and that the staff member will go beyond her duty to help Annie with things, such as when her grandma died and she wanted a commemorative plant for the garden:

Annie: But if I've needed her and she knows I need her, she's always been there for me. If I've ever gone up to her and I've scared myself when I've self-harmed or I've done something that bad that I don't think I can handle it myself, I can always go up to her and say 'Look, this is what's happened.' Or if I've wanted to phone my mum or whatever, or I've needed her to get in touch with my mum, she's always gone and done what she's, got the number or asked if I can phone her. It's like with the plant for my grandma and stuff, it were her who actually fought for me to get the plant and stuff.

(Interview, client, LSU)

The themes running throughout these responses are that staff were offering much emotional support, but also they were being asked to do things *for* the clients, because the clients were not allowed to do these things for themselves. I saw lots of staff being asked to do things such as bring items, switch over the TV, telephone people, write something down, and these things were due to the clients being unable to access a certain space or move between spaces. Women valued these gestures of assistance, but one of the main problems with this was that staff had other demands on their time and may be seen to 'put off' the person by saying they would do something later. This is something I also saw regularly, which staff member Iona explains here:

Iona: They get you to do things either by being really nice or really horrible. But do you not think that's because of the way we set our role up? For a lot of those women, because we're the jailors, we're inviting that 'I want I want' thing, because we're denying people it. Whereas if we put the responsibility on the women themselves, [saying to them] 'It's your responsibility to manage your own cigarettes,' whatever. We still dominate people.

(Interview, qualified staff)

Iona was commenting on the aspect of the staff role which often involves containing and controlling the clients. Many of the staff mentioned this as a difficult part of their job, balancing the two aspects of their role, therapy and containment, and how to do this. If *trust* is an essential aspect of the therapeutic relationship as discussed in the literature, then it is going to be very difficult to achieve when staff are accountable to the management as well as clients. It seemed on Unit C that the requirements of management and clients were necessarily conflicting, as management had a duty to control and contain clients.

Negative influences on the staff/client relationship

Most of the staff told me examples of good relationships with clients. They spoke about the sense of achievement they experience when they can see 'progress' in a client [notions of progression will be explored in Chapter 6]. However, they also talked about factors that can damage the staff/client relationship.

When a client has less perceived cognitive ability, they can be considered to have less control over their behaviour, and as needing more support. This is evidenced by the excerpt from fieldnotes here:

> The staff member tells me that Tara has less cognitive ability than the others, so is not as manipulative, which may be why the staff have more time for her.
> (Fieldnotes, LSU)

Although Tara was someone who self-harmed severely, as she was considered to be less 'able' than others, she was sometimes treated with more regard and understanding than other clients. This could be analysed in terms of power differentials on the ward; staff were there to contain clients as well as support them to progress through the service. Clients who were considered 'manipulative' were perceived to be resisting the rules intentionally (Nathan et al., 2007). More about these struggles will be discussed in the next chapter which is concerned with power and control on the secure unit.

When a client is aggressive with a staff member, this can undermine their relationship, especially when there is a situation where restraint or seclusion has to be used. If the client is aggressive with a staff member who thinks that they have a good relationship, this can cause feelings of failure and distress in staff members, as reported by Fish and Culshaw (2005). Some staff can manage this aggression, by using humour and offering 'face saving' alternatives (see Duperouzel, 2008), as Iona pointed out below, that humour and patience in the face of aggression could enable relationships:

Iona: One of the first things she said to me she came over, she said 'Iona' – she whispered this in my ear, she had a good look round first of all. She said in a very menacing way, 'There's little voices in my head telling me to attack you.' And to appear tough and not be intimidated because you do put this facade on just to protect yourself, my reply was '(Name), this little voice is telling you to bugger off.' And she laughed just like that. She laughed and that was the start of a really interesting relationship.

Iona went on to describe how her positive relationship with this client worked to reduce her aggression; however, this relationship was looked on with suspicion by other staff:

Iona: My attitude towards her was very upbeat and very OK. I was never negative towards her, if she couldn't do something I didn't say it in a negative way. And the relationship was very different between them two [staff members] and her because they'd had all the aggression and I'd never had aggression. We'd have a laugh to be honest, we'd laugh and joke and I think there was an element of – what's the difference? [They thought that I] must be doing something for her that I shouldn't be doing. Because there's that punitive role, they'd have a lot of animosity for her because of all the battles they'd had with her. Their attitude towards her was very different than mine, whereas I'd always had a very positive relationship with her.

(Female qualified staff)

Iona's comment shows that aggression arises in a relational context, and importantly, that a positive staff/client relationship can work to reduce aggression. Other staff members were suspicious of the relationship and assumed that Iona was being unprofessional, showing that staff/client relationships are subjected to regulation in the unit. As explained in the descriptions of BPD earlier, this can be described as 'splitting' and perceived as a result of pathology of the (female) client.

Concepts of the client's index offence (the reason why they were in a secure service) also negatively affected relationships between clients and staff. Although some of the staff told me that they tried not to read about a client's past before spending time with them and getting to know them, to avoid the offence being their first impression of the person (Shattell et al., 2007), clients' offences did feature in the minds of staff when they seem at odds with the client's demeanour, for example:

> Dawn tells me that Jane is a very likeable person who is happy to go along with things, however, she remains constantly wary of her because of her index offence which was violent and serious. It's almost as though she thinks that Jane may show her true colours at any time.
>
> *(Fieldnotes)*

If Dawn is 'wary' of the client in this case, this will affect her relationship with her. Trust in inpatient settings is described as an essential basis for the therapeutic relationship, and despite the literature mainly focussing on clients trusting staff, Langley and Klopper (2005:30) define relationships as 'feedback loops', where the behaviour of each person affects and is affected. They point out that only by being trusted can a person learn to trust himself or herself.

When a client self-harms, this can also affect the therapeutic relationship (Fish and Duperouzel, 2008). Here, Bella talked about becoming trusted more now that she has stopped self-harming:

Bella: But I haven't done it for three weeks, which I'm very, very proud of myself. I'm very proud of myself and so are the staff. And they're now starting to trust me they are, because I've a little box, you know in craft, and the lady in art and crafts said "don't look because I'm putting a rib-bon on it", and I just looked up and I said, 'Right I can't have one, because I tied ligatures.' She said thanks for telling her – 'I'll cut it into pieces.' So that's what I said, I am getting better Rebecca about telling them about myself or why I'm doing things. But I do occasionally do it.

(Interview, client, MSU)

Bella described owning up to staff that she might tie a ligature if she was allowed a piece of ribbon. She also described feeling more trusted because she had not self-harmed for three weeks. This suggests that self-harming on the unit is seen as breaking the rules, and by self-harming, Bella feels as though she might be letting the staff down.

Many of the qualified staff would discuss problems with the relationship in terms of attachment theory (Bowlby, 2005) and although this model seemed to provide a helpful way for staff to come to terms with women's current presenta-tion, it did not seem to offer any way of dealing with problems in the future. Adele discussed the way she thought about attachment here:

Adele: You often hear staff say things like, 'Well, I gave her all the attention and then at the end of the day she had an incident anyway', that sort of thing, 'What was that all about?' And that's really a chance [for quali-fied staff] to explain 'Well that was about the fact that she knew you were about to go home and didn't want to lose that closeness. She was attached to you for that particular shift, had been following you around all day, you'd been giving her loads of support, but she knew that you had to go home and it was her way of saying 'I don't want you to go.'

(Interview, qualified staff)

Although the use of attachment theory seems a positive step as it encouraged viewing the woman's behaviour in the context of their past experiences, it still meant that close therapeutic relationships were framed as inherently problematic. Rather than looking to the regime and power structures in the organisation (as I will discuss in the next chapter), or at staff's own attachment patterns in a rela-tional sense, the centre of analysis is again focussed on the client.

The theme which runs through the concept of staff/client relationships in this study is trust. Trust works both ways and is described as central to the therapeutic relationship. According to Langley and Klopper (2005), essential conditions for the development of trust in a staff member are availability, honesty and confi-dentiality, being able to listen and try to understand, and helping the client to feel safe emotionally and physically. The clients in this study felt that the need to be trusted was as important as being able to trust, as I will also show in the next chapter.

Opportunities for the staff/client relationship to be more one of friendship and mutual support were being missed due to the power imbalance between staff and clients and because positive relationships were considered to hold clients back in their rehabilitation. This was recognised by staff as part of the contradictory requirements of care and control. Within this type of relationship, there is likely to be a large imbalance of power, where attempts to spend time with staff will seem like attention-seeking behaviour.

It is worthwhile noting that outside of professional jargon (such as 'care plan', 'person-centred care' etc.) staff did not use the word 'care' to describe their work or relationships with clients (Morris, 1993; Potier, 1993; Walmsley, 1996). They used words such as 'empathy' and 'support', even 'friendship', which I would suggest reflects the nature of the relationship and the type of work (Thomas, 1993). 'Care' was used by staff when talking about physical aspects of nursing, for example when Monica talked about caring for people with physical needs, and also when discussing how clients felt about one another, as I shall show.

I did see many examples of good relationships between staff and clients, and Iona's illustration shows that positive relationships can reduce aggressive behaviour. However, the way female clients are described in the service as 'manipulative', and conceptions of behaviour as related to the person rather than the context, may damage these fragile relationships. This is likely to be exacerbated when staff are stressed and short of time which was often the case on the wards when I was there. The concept of positive relationships as holding clients back, as I will show in Chapter 6, is further damaging (McMillan and Aiyegbusi, 2008). I would suggest more focus and regard to be placed on secure or safe staff/client relationships, for them to be comprehended and described as a 'supportive alliance' and a base for future progression.

Family relationships – 'I'm just thinking of her today'

Families provide much support for learning disabled people who live in the community; they help with stressful times and can offer an extraordinary amount of assistance in daily life (Goldberg et al., 2003; Roffman, 2000; Rolph et al., 2006; Tuffrey-Wijne et al., 2009). Good family relationships are described as enhancing self-image and resilience and caring skills in people (Walmsley, 1993; Morrison and Cosden, 1997; Nunkoosing and John, 1997; Knox and Bigby, 2007). Families were extremely important to the women on Unit C. When women talked about their families, it was often in terms of looking forward to seeing them, worrying about things happening to them, and wishing they could be with their families to help them in one way or another.

Rebecca: So what do you not like about living here?
Sarah: Being away from your family, at Christmas time, locked away. What I do like about it is when we have a home visit, that's what I like about

it, but what I don't like is when you're just locked here at Christmas time and everything.

(Interview, client, MSU)

As found in other research projects, clients at Unit C often felt that they did not see their family often enough (Goodwin, 1999; Wood et al., 2008) and this was described as frustrating. This might be especially significant due to learning disabled people often living at home with their families into their adult lives. Despite policy urging that people access services as near to their families as possible (Reed, 1994), it seemed that some of the women were far from home which was detrimental to their family visits:

Rebecca: What about the weekends?
Katrina: Crap. The only thing that's good is that I see my mum. She comes all the way from [town – about 2 hours' drive away]. I go on home visits to try and save her from driving.
Rebecca: Do you have to take staff with you?
Katrina: Yes two staff.
Rebecca: I imagine that's quite hard to organise. Is it?
Katrina: I haven't been on a home visit for a while.

(Interview, client, LSU)

All except one of the women I spoke to received visits from their family or partner, and some were allowed to visit home with the support of staff for the occasional weekend, with frequency being dependent on Home Office approval. What they did at the visit depended on the client's guidelines, for example some families could take their member out to town or to the Unit cafeteria. Most of the women told me however, that they mainly sat in the visiting room to talk to their families, accompanied by a member of staff,

Rebecca: Do your family come and see you?
Lorna: Yes, we just sit in this room and chat.
Rebecca: How long for?
Lorna: Two hours max.
Rebecca: And do you like it when they come?
Lorna: Yes.
Rebecca: How often do they come?
Lorna: Not often about once a month.

(Interview, client, MSU)

Three of the women were worried about family members who were in ill health. They found it distressing that they could not visit them:

Bella: [My Mum is very ill and] she says she doesn't want no birthday presents or Christmas presents because she doesn't know how long she's going to be [alive], so I said I'd get her a little cuddly teddy so she can have a teddy with her. I'm just thinking of her today. It's getting harder though because I'm just waiting for the phone call do you know what I mean?

(Interview, client, LSU)

Despite these desires, it seemed clear that much of the violence and abuse in the women's pasts had come from family members, and staff naturally had to find a way to protect clients from those people. Much of staff's discussion about families was negative, they seemed to take on the role of mediator, for example:

> Lorna has been writing a letter in her room. Candice tells me (with Lorna's agreement) that Lorna has been having some problems with her family and she has been supporting her to write a letter to them telling them how she feels, and making it known that she will not give them money any more.
>
> *(Fieldnotes)*

It was clear that staff in the service were supportive in maintaining family links, with phone calls to family evident in the evenings and some discussion about both staff and clients' families on the wards. Phone times were allocated to clients on the LSU and they could use the telephone sited in the kitchen to make calls in the evening. In the MSU there was a mobile phone which clients could take into their room. There was no discussion, however, about how family were included in any meetings or consultation about the women's care and no reference to clients' families in staff interviews (although I did not ask about this specifically and this could have been related to confidentiality concerns).

Clients spoke about how important family was to them, and families formed a fundamental part of people's conceptions about their future. Even though many people had negative relationships with some family members, they often spoke about *other* family members as significant and their relationships with them as positive.

Peer relationships – 'We've managed to lean on each other'

Almost all of the research which mentions relationships on inpatient units focusses only on the therapeutic relationship between staff and clients. Clients' relationships with each other are discussed occasionally within literature which explores client satisfaction with services and papers which discuss the 'ward milieu'. The reported significance of peer relationships differs greatly in these accounts; Goffman (1961) in *Asylums* describes little solidarity and support between clients, and Bressington (2011), for example, observed that peer support had very little to do with how satisfied clients were with their inpatient stay. Opposing views come from the participants in Thomas et al.'s (2002) study with psychiatric inpatients. They reported that universally, peer-administered 'therapy' was the most beneficial aspect of hospitalisation, which usually took place in the smoke room away from staff. This sentiment was similar to Howard et al.'s (2001) study, again on a psychiatric ward, where participants rated their satisfaction with opportunities to talk with other patients as greater than any other aspect of their hospital experience. Support groups such as the Hearing Voices Network are being established in England, where service users can describe their experiences and understandings about their conditions in a supportive atmosphere (Hornstein, 2013).

McWade (2014) found that relationships with peers in an English NHS 'Arts for Mental Health' service were very important to service users. Her participants said that these relationships enabled them to feel less isolated, and to realise that there were people with whom they had some shared experiences and understanding. They linked meaningful relationships with feelings of joy and excitement, and pathways to recovery. According to Wolfson et al. (2009), clients with mental health conditions who are recovering are able to help others and this should be encouraged by staff; however, they also emphasise that peer relationships are not always about support, people experiencing different conditions are 'thrown together' which can result in hostility, bullying and harassment.

The Unit does have comprehensive policies that provide guidance on safeguarding vulnerable people and supporting personal relationships. These make reference to and are a reflection of national policy; however, national guidance on safeguarding, such as the Department of Health document *No Secrets* (Department of Health, 2000) has been criticised for emphasising the vulnerability of people rather than recognising and encouraging their strengths and capabilities. Consequently, this can result in staff focussing on 'protection' rather than 'choice' (Braye et al., 2010), which is an issue in this study. Critically, the call for more appropriate policy that takes into account individual needs has been made (Dein and Williams, 2008; Fyson and Kitson, 2010; Fulford and Cobigo, 2016), and the issue of relationships on Unit C adds to the discussion about the extent to which individual needs are taken into account.

Although I did see some supportive relationships between clients, by far the largest interview theme relating to clients' relationships with each other was conflict; people talking about arguments and fights with others. When clients are forced to live in close proximity with other peoples who are not of their choosing, spending large parts of their day in their company, this often causes problems. This was especially the case when clients were obliged to remain in the same physical area for surveillance reasons. Even though other clients may not be designated to need this level of observation, due to staffing regulations, they had to remain in the same spaces. When I was spending time on the LSU, two clients who lived in the same flat were arguing after previously being good friends:

> Teresa is having a cigarette outside and I am with her. Elaine comes through the door and says, 'Say anything about me and I'll smash your head in.' Teresa's bottom lip wobbles and she has a very sad face. It is time for me to go, I ask Teresa, 'Will you be OK?' She replies, 'No.' I ask her, 'Are you scared?' She replies, 'Yes.' She goes inside and says she doesn't want her food. I ask her if she will eat it if I stay and she agrees. The staff member gives me some background to this exchange, she says that Elaine has lived

alone for years and she is very outspoken if she's annoyed about something. Both women have been avoiding each other and not eating because of this. They got on really well at first, they have similar ages, similar interests. Teresa tells me it is because Elaine kept wanting the sweets that Teresa's husband had brought her. When she has gone, the staff member tells me that she also thinks Elaine is jealous of the things that Teresa's husband brings for her. Although Elaine gets to go home and see her mum, she always has to take something, her mum never gives Elaine anything. The staff have tried to explain to her that everyone is different and has different amounts of stuff, but she hasn't accepted it.

(Fieldnotes, LSU)

Jealousy was attributed as the cause for many problems and was a recurring theme when discussing clients' arguments, as pointed out by staff member Stewart:

Stewart: The main thing again, is – and I keep repeating myself – the relationships, 90%, just to pluck a figure – of incidents on the ward are usually revolving around high-expressed emotions of jealousy or things like that really. Someone'll get a visit which will annoy the other person because they haven't had a visit for maybe two weeks, or someone will get down and things like that really. Certainly the jealousy between clients is big, certainly when you're dealing with people with personality disorders, they might seem to go out of their way to cause friction and light the touch paper then retreat. They seem to enjoy someone else losing it because of what they've said to wind them up.

(Interview, staff member, qualified)

Stewart attributed some of the jealousy on the Unit to the behaviour of particular women, indicating that feelings of jealousy are not always unavoidable but brought about on purpose. Annie, a client gave me an example of conflict which could be considered to be due to jealousy, here:

Annie: And I'd been nagging and nagging and nagging for ages to go and get this MP3 player, and Tilly knew I wanted this MP3 player, and my mum bought it with a message that my (late) grandma apparently wrote to me saying goodbye and all this sort of stuff. And she put mine and my grandma's favourite song on this MP3 player. And to cut a long story short it was in my bedroom and I'd hid it purposely because of the way that she was, and she went in my bedroom and she hunted high and low for my MP3 player, she smashed it to smithereens and then was singing the song at the top of her voice on the corridor but doing it to the point where I could hear it.

Rebecca: How did she get in your room?

Annie: Because my door wasn't locked at that time. And she went in, smashed it up and put it on a chair so when I went in I could see it. But no one had actually heard Tilly turn round and say, 'Ha I've smashed it up, she's never going to remember her grandma again.'

Rebecca: That's terrible, what happened?

Annie: I was basically devastated, I went to the night staff, threw it at the night staff and said 'Look what I have to put up with!' and they said, 'Well you shouldn't have left it in your room you should have locked it up.' But it was two night staff that was on that night that love Tilly to bits, they'll go up to her hug her and hold her hands, if she cuts up they look after her and make sure she's alright.

(Interview, client, LSU)

Annie suggested that Tilly was jealous of her MP3 player, but then she also implied that she herself was jealous of Tilly's relationships with the staff. This, along with my previous observations suggests that there was conflict between them already and Tilly may have been using the MP3 player as retaliation for what has happened previously. Annie was using the MP3 player as a symbol of her continued relationship with her family, and as a way to explain her behaviour in response to its destruction. The importance of material items as symbols of relationship is described by Parrott (2005) who points out how these items can be experienced as interpersonal connections with family and future. It seems that both staff and clients used a rationale of 'jealousy' about relationships and material items as an accepted way to explain disputes which may have much more complex origins. These explanations are unhelpful and generate further arguments.

Because of the amount of conflict between clients, many discussions about activities and visits to different areas of the unit included concerns of compatibility. Problems arose when two clients were seen to have had a long-term conflict and one of the clients had been moved because of this. Often, time was spent deciding who could go where and with whom; however, it was often evident that women were living with other women that they clashed with in some way, for example:

Adele: But in relation to [living on the unit], making people worse, I think there's probably inevitably a sense that people who're distressed living with other people who're distressed, it's not ideal is it really? Compatibility issues are huge aren't they here? And in places like this, and I think because we're often at full capacity you have people living together who, for all sorts of reasons, see each other, when they were living together they see themselves in the other person and it's almost unbearable.

(Interview staff member, qualified)

Adele's answer implies that conflicts between women were as a result of them seeing 'themselves in the other person'. Research in the mental health field shows that people who have similar issues are able to offer coping strategies and hope for the future to each other. It is interesting that Adele considered this to be a cause of problems, rather than contextual issues on the wards such as the lack of privacy.

Despite the level of conflict between clients, there were many positive relationships being played out on the ward. I saw evidence of clients helping and supporting each other, cheering each other up and offering consolation in bad times. I also saw examples of clients offering ways of coping to other clients, such as suggesting ways of thinking about the future and family to keep them going, Annie pinpoints this in her statement:

Annie: We've managed to lean on each other and pick each other up and when one's down, the other one's alright so whoever's alright manages to pick the other person up.

(Interview, client, LSU)

I saw Marion and another client helping and reassuring each other often, during times of distress for both of them. Here, she explains about their relationship in an interview:

Marion: We just sit and talk, (name) very very helpful, she's very very good to me is (name). She helps me put my necklaces on for me because I have problems getting them on myself so she helps me.

(Interview, client, LSU)

When women were described (and described themselves) as 'unwell', it indicated that they were going through a time of particular distress and might self-harm or act aggressively towards staff or other clients. During these times it was common for them to turn to each other for support. Kate told me about her relationship with an older woman on her flat:

Kate: I'm not allowed to see my Mum. So we've got a nice lady on here called (name). She's um, she's my mum. She says, 'I'm your adoptive mother now,' and she looks after me in any way possible. Like before she said if I told her I was going to self-harm, she'd go straight to the staff, she wouldn't try and stop me, she'd just say 'Look Kate don't.' But if I was determined, she wouldn't intervene but she'd go and tell staff before I had chance to do it. So erm yes she's good with me.

Rebecca: And what kind of things do you do together?

Kate: Oh we sit, we chat, we read magazines together, sometimes we watch films together. We just do all sorts really, board games, colouring, all sorts we do together.

(Interview, client, LSU)

Kate describes a supportive relationship which is played out in terms of a mother/daughter dynamic. The older client she describes as her 'Mum' used to self-harm but managed to stop, and now she helps Kate by summoning staff when she feels like self-harming.

A number of clients pointed out to me that they were not encouraged to have close relationships with other clients. Here, Helen explained that clients as well as staff could get moved when a good relationship had been established:

Rebecca: What about another client, do you have a good friend here?

Helen: Not really, I've been told not to get too close to people because you end up losing them or something, or they end up getting moved or something like that. So there's no point having a relationship because they might get moved one day and then you've lost that relationship.

Rebecca: So you're trying your best not to get close to anyone?

Helen: Well I get close to them but there's only a certain point now that will happen, because it's happened too many times before, I'm getting on well with staff and they get moved.

Rebecca: And how do you feel when they get moved?

Helen: I think that it's my fault but I've been told it's not my fault.

(Interview, client, MSU)

Although it seems as though Helen was repeating something she had been told often by staff, that staff moves were not her fault, it seems that she still felt responsible for them. While it is not clear why staff were moved from working with Helen, as I show elsewhere (Harker-Longton and Fish, 2002) it is extremely distressing for clients when people are moved and relationships break down as a result. Client moves were also described as distressing by some clients in this study. I saw two clients preparing to move wards and witnessed the tears and sadness from other clients, as well as women feeling upset and worried that others seemed to be progressing but they themselves were not moving on. In this example, Annie pointed out why she was not encouraged to meet up with another client after moving:

Annie: [We don't meet up] because they said the relationship was getting too personal for Jane, because she is, she is ill but she needed that 1:1 with me because she knew I was the only person that she could trust, from day one I'd been there with her, I'd been there when she were cutting up and [graphic descriptions of self-harm incidents and expressions of distress]. I just used to sit there with her and none of the staff would go anywhere near because they were too scared. I'm like 'No just let me be with her I'm alright.' And she just used to come out and get hold of me, yes I'd lose my rag with her I'd shout and scream at her and she'd just take it. But anyone else did it she'd lose her rag with them. And it got to the point where we'd built up a good relationship with her and we all worked really well with her and then everyone turned on me then, they didn't want her to know me. So then Jane started hurting herself then because she felt sorry for me, so it's all gone different.

(Interview, client, LSU)

There are a number of things happening here. Annie said that she was told that her relationship was getting 'too personal' with the other client, which may have been the case, with Annie suggesting the client's self-harm was because of her. However, Annie also mentioned that the relationship was of benefit for some time previously. It is unclear why the staff were discouraging this supportive relationship since the client had moved wards. Annie told me that she had asked to see this client many times but this had not happened.

This discouragement is referred to in literature; Clements et al.'s (1995) research in a learning disability challenging behaviour service, for example, illustrates how services promote independence and autonomy and devote very little attention to supportive relationships. They put this down to the elevation of 'independent functioning' (Clements et al., 1995:429) as the most important goal of services, due to the style of care being focussed on traditionally masculine values:

> The goal is to help those who use services develop towards some notion of (lonely) self sufficiency. Loneliness and the absence of friendship are often remarked upon. Yet services do little to address this issue – how often do those who use services exercise any control over something as basic as who they live with?
>
> (Clements et al., 1995:428)

Clements et al. further comment on the ideology within services, as the 'individual as the focus for change' and point out the absence of focus on *relationships* and *feelings* in services (Clements et al., 1995:429). Becker (1997:98) puts this down to the fact that 'the glorification of autonomous functioning has been achieved by excluding a sense of relatedness from the pantheon of cultural values' in society. She describes how 'effectiveness and competence' are valued and only achievable by individual action, that women are socialised to define their identity based on relational experiences and this is then pathologised due to the implicit connection of weakness with dependence.

Although clients' relationships on Unit C were complex and it is impossible to make judgements about them here, it does seem that more focus should be placed on understanding and supporting relationships, rather than mainly treating them as negative. In my time at the unit it seemed that whether or not supportive relationships were accepted depended on staff's judgement of the relationship. The organisation was making moves to remedy the issue of conflict between clients; during my time on the unit 'community meetings' were being introduced, as Adele described:

Adele: The staff support sessions on the women's flat for the medium secure unit is not around one client, it's around all of them and the dynamics of them all living together and how difficult that is, and it's basically about the psychological treatment service supporting the staff that look after those five women together. It's happening now on the LSU as well, there are staff support sessions over there for various people.

(Interview, qualified staff)

Although Adele was mainly focussing on staff support to enable women to live together, this was a step in the right direction. Nevertheless, Adele was still framing clients' relationships with each other in a negative sense, as 'difficult'.

Despite all this negativity, Jackie had great things to say about the 'care' that women can offer to each other, particularly in terms of being part of a group:

Jackie: [Women], they have a huge capacity to care for other people and each other and so many want to work with animals, or older people or children. And I think there's something about when you get them together as well and you empower them and you give them a voice. So rather than competing with each other in a negative way for what they feel is a scarce resource in terms of care, they can care about each other and when that happens it's brilliant. They're really wise as well; they can give each other sometimes really good advice. They can't always follow it themselves, because they can't always see. And that's great because it's not relying necessarily on the staff for all the advice, but it comes from within them.

(Interview, qualified staff)

Jackie's powerful words are advocating the encouragement of women as caring for each other, rather than competing with each other. Despite the constant threat of conflict, clients found ways to maintain supportive relationships and help each other by offering coping strategies when they perceive they are needed, for example suggesting that the client 'think of their family' or 'think about the future'. This is described by some researchers as 'peer administered therapy' as I have mentioned, which often takes place away from the gaze of staff (Thomas et al., 2002; Shattell et al., 2008) and can be more beneficial to some clients than any other intervention (Thomas et al., 2002; Happell, 2008). A significant theme in the disability studies literature is one of 'interdependence', acknowledging that nobody is fully independent and therefore this should not be an expectation (Walmsley, 1993; Carnaby, 1998; Reindal, 1999; Lloyd, 2001; Garland-Thomson, 2003; White et al., 2010). The importance of mutually supportive relationships within disability studies and the mental health literature is clear, and I would argue that this concept of interdependence should be the way forward for everyone at Unit C.

Sexual violence

During analysis, I found that sexual violence emerged as one of the most significant themes. More than half of the clients I interviewed disclosed experiences of abuse as children, or sexual violence as adults, even though I did not question them directly about this, for example, Bonnie told me:

Bonnie: I mean me and my mum have never had a good relationship. From the age of 2 till I was 8 I was in and out of care, then when I was 8 I had to give evidence against my brother, my uncle, my dad and my next door neighbour in court, about abusing me.

(Interview, client, LSU)

In her interview it seems Kate attributes her mental state that contributed to fire-setting to the fact that she was abused as a child, and she pointed out the lasting damage that the abuse had on her:

Kate: I was um, I was very, very, very disturbed (pause) because of all the sexual abuse from my dad and that, I was really really, I was disturbed in the head, I guess you could say I was a psycho back in them days. Because I actually set fire to my own house, whilst a member of staff were upstairs and I didn't even know I done it.

(Interview, client, LSU)

Another service user, Ellie recalls the sexual violence she experienced in a home she lived in previously. Here, she expresses just how much the experience affects her currently:

Ellie: It's still in my head at night . . . I've never talked to her about it because I was too scared to tell anyone, but it's all coming in my mind and I want to get it off my mind
Rebecca: Did you not feel like you could say 'no, I don't want you to do that to me'?
Ellie: He wouldn't let me, he went like that to my face in my bedroom [holds face tight].
Rebecca: So is this why you're concerned about men now?
Ellie: Yeah. I won't even give my dad a hug because I'm too scared to hug anyone, but I'm trying to build that confidence up between me and my dad to hug him, because I used to hug dad before [this experience], but I won't hug him now.

(Interview, client, LSU)

In my interview data there were a number of stories about sexual violence within services; Ellie's story concerned a staff member in a previous service, and other women described sexual assaults from other clients, male and female, identifying that women are not always safe when living in an inpatient services. For example, Kate also experienced sexual violence when living in an inpatient service; here she describes evocatively how she felt when she was raped in the grounds of that service:

Rebecca: Were you scared? Did you not scream?
Kate: Yes I did but I couldn't move because in a way I was paralysed so I couldn't move but after it happened I come back, didn't say anything for a couple of days and staff knew sommat were up and they said 'Has sommat happened?' And I just burst into tears and told them what happened.
Rebecca: Did you have to have a pregnancy test?
Kate: Yes I had to get pregnancy tested and then I had to go for um (long pause)

Rebecca: Did they take swabs?

Kate: Yes, swabs and internal examinations, swabs.

Rebecca: Oh you poor thing.

Kate: The worst thing, the worst thing about it was, I was raped by a male in [service] whilst I'm supposed to be safe but it was my own fault because I did say I was [at work] when I weren't. But then when I went for my swab, there was a man doing it because there was no female available. And they said, 'You can come back at a later date if you want a female but chances are the evidence won't be there so we need to get it while it's fresh.' So I just bit my tongue and let him get it.

(Interview, service user)

What this narrative explicitly tells us is that clients are not always safe even within services, and police treatment of learning disabled women who have been raped can be inappropriate and ill conceived (see also Petersilia, 2000). Worryingly, Kate felt that the incident was her 'own fault.'

Interviews with staff members indicate that staff did understand that women had experienced sexual violence in their past, and many of them pointed out that they see the challenging behaviour of the women in terms of past experiences of abuse. For example, Iona said:

Iona: It was all so obvious when you sit and listen to people's stories this is why people behave this way, um some very light-bulb moments in my head. If you've never experienced abuse, you've never experienced abuse. Not just abuse as a woman but abuse as a vulnerable woman, no matter how gobby [outspoken] and confident they seem, they are all very very vulnerable. From very poor backgrounds a lot of them, starved of support and love really.

(Interview, qualified staff)

Iona, a professional nurse who has worked with women for 25 years, points out that women have had bad experiences in their past, and less than ideal backgrounds. The way women are described as 'vulnerable' as a result of this, however, can result in the focus being on the woman and her personal history rather than her current circumstances (Hollomotz, 2011).

Regulated behaviour

Although the unit forbids sexual activity with the rationale that all spaces are public, my observations established that intimate relationships were played out on the unit. Indeed there were attempts to control the types of behaviour on the wards which are single sex, as can be seen from my fieldnotes:

On the (Perspex covered) noticeboard there is a typed A4 sheet named 'Conduct on the ward.' It has a list of things that clients are allowed to do, for example 'Clients can sit with one hand on another client's knee. Clients can greet each other with a peck on the cheek.' The last item is 'No swearing.' When I ask a member of staff if they are able to have physical contact with others in the privacy of their room, I am told that because it is a secure unit, all spaces are classed as public, so this is not possible.

(Fieldnotes)

Men and women were not allowed in each other's living accommodation; they encountered each other during day services, in the grounds, and sometimes during social activities in the evening. In these spaces they were able to play pool, listen to music and buy snacks from a vending machine. Staff concerns focussed on protecting women from mixing with men who were offenders. For example, Karen, a qualified member of staff, told me during an interview that:

Karen: They're just told that relationships are not allowed. They're not allowed. But again these women that say they're going out with someone, they're not told the history or the index offence and it's very difficult that because if they knew, then . . . Mind you some of them if they knew anyway it wouldn't make any difference because that's what they've grown up with isn't it? And some of these women will always end up with [that type of man] they will bless them, they will. Because that's all they know and they're so vulnerable, they're targeted aren't they?

(Interview, qualified staff)

Karen's comment reflects the popular discourse that some women tend to repeat patterns from their past by choosing partners similar to those who have violated them. She suggested that women are not able to make informed decisions about prospective partners because they are not party to the same knowledge as staff about the person's offence. Jackie, however, another qualified member of staff, acknowledged the role of the organisation in this type of situation:

Jackie: But then there's also something about not putting them in the situations that maybe re-enact situations that they've been in in the past in terms of abuse or being at risk of men. Or perhaps in terms of their behaviour when they've become around men that they put themselves at risk for all sorts of reasons.

(Interview, qualified staff)

Jackie's narrative is particularly relevant to the discourse which is used around women and vulnerability. She described women putting themselves at risk, 'for all sorts of reasons', emphasising as Karen did, that women ultimately end up recreating abusive situations from the past by being attracted to the same sort of person in the present. After all, this is with what some of them are most familiar. Although this discourse points to areas where therapy and education are needed, it is still situating the burden of responsibility as within the victim.

The lack of information given to women about sexual relationships may be a symptom of the lack of consideration given to women's sexuality, as illustrated in my fieldnotes:

> There was some discussion about the male clients and their medication, apparently there have been complaints about medication ruining their 'sex lives.' I enquire whether they are allowed a sex life in the unit. The staff member says, 'Yes, with themselves.' This causes me to think afterwards that I have heard talk about men's sexual needs, but no such talk about women. The lack of privacy offered to certain women who are subjected to 'special observations', where staff members have to watch them constantly in case they try to self-harm, should highlight these concerns.
>
> *(Fieldnotes)*

Importantly, though the women were not considered as 'needing' sexual gratification, if they did want to participate in sexual activity they were sometimes described as promiscuous:

> Linda tells me about a client, who in the past has inserted items into her vagina. She tells me that once, a long time ago, she was caught having sex with a male service user in the laundry room, they'd managed to initiate penetrative sex in the very short time before the member of staff entered the room. Linda tells me that the woman is 'very promiscuous.'
>
> *(Fieldnotes)*

These two examples suggest that sometimes women are not expected to want or need sexual experiences, and those who show that they are interested in sex are at risk of being seen as deviant. The regulation of women's sexuality was related to the perceived risk posed by male offenders residing at the unit.

Resistance

It was very difficult for people to meet potential partners on Unit C. This was seen by the women as very important, even in light of their abusive pasts. Although, women who were married were allowed visits from their partners (without privacy for sexual encounters, however). Clients were often unsure what behaviour was 'allowed' within sexual relationships, or even the reasons why such behaviour was controlled. Despite this, there were many efforts to remain in contact with potential partners. For example, Helen told me in an interview:

Helen: It is difficult, but there is someone that I like on the ward next door. But because we're not allowed to write, well someone said we're allowed to write letters and they sometimes say we're not and that's why it's not got any further because we don't know where we stand – if we're allowed to write letters or if we're not. So we need to talk to our case managers or our key workers and get it checked to see what we're allowed to do.

(Interview, client, MSU)

The service had decided to segregate some of the women and men based on individual risk assessment due to an incident that happened prior to my fieldwork. Only certain people were allowed to socialise on a 'mixed' basis. Women were not clear what was the reason for this, and believed that it was because some people were having sex and this was somehow 'dangerous' for example as Kate told me:

Kate: Yes, because if we're on group, day services bring us back, day staff drop us off and day services staff bring us back. But they've split the sessions haven't they? Strictly female, strictly male or mixed. And the ones that can't be mixed, they're saying that on the way back we're not allowed to talk to any of the lads or the lads aren't allowed to talk to any of the women on the way back and if we do try to say hello, they sort of like separate us! And it's not right, it shouldn't be happening because it makes us feel like we've done something wrong that we haven't – it's all because of four different clients. All this has changed because of four clients having sex in the toilets at the club, the poly tunnels in the gardens. This is all because of four clients this. No-one else has done anything, it's all because of them four clients.

Rebecca: Is that what happened?

Kate: Yes, it is because of four clients. One set were boyfriend and girl-friend and the other set were boyfriend and girlfriend and um, they were basically going into the club toilets whenever they could, having sex or the poly tunnels whenever they could and they got caught on all the occasions. And it was actually the Valentine's party that got cancelled first because of it. The staff felt it wasn't enough time to safeguard everybody because the party only got cancelled three days before it was due to start. So there weren't enough time to figure out who was dangerous and who weren't. So they had to stop it completely. And I did see him for a couple of weeks after that at the club, and then it just went.

Rebecca: Can you write letters to each other?

Kate: Yes, but we don't really like doing that because it's not right. We shouldn't have to just write letters we should be able to see each other. And he's getting upset about it, I'm getting upset about it [sigh].

                                                              (Interview, client, LSU)

Clearly men and women were being segregated based on the actions of others; however, many of the women did not know the reasons for this segregation and specifically pointed this out as not equating to community life, as shown here:

Rebecca: Would you prefer it if there were men there?

Teresa: Yes. It's not normal though is it? Just women, you wouldn't have that in the community would you? How are you supposed to get to the community when they're doing this?

Rebecca: Why do you think they're doing it?

Teresa: I don't know. It's not normal life that.

Rebecca:	No, and what about the club, would you go if there was men there?
Teresa:	Yes, some, there's mixed sessions and there's all female sessions and there's all male sessions. But that's not normal life, just females is it?

(Interview, service user)

Teresa had a clear idea about what 'normal life' was like. By equating sex segregation with incarceration, Teresa felt that the rule was punitive. Despite this type of regulation on the unit, still women managed to establish relationships with potential partners as Katrina told me:

Rebecca:	OK, I know you've got a boyfriend here, how often do you get to see him?
Katrina:	Every other Thursday, at the canteen. We're engaged. [shows me her engagement ring]. He gave it me last Thursday. He said will I marry him and I said yes.
Rebecca:	When are you going to get married?
Katrina:	When we get out of here.

(Interview, client, LSU)

Rather than having to rely on the club to see her boyfriend, Katrina was able to see him at the canteen, but this situation was dependent on staffing. It seems that the regulations were being interpreted in different ways depending on the individual, for example despite people being told they should not have physical contact, they found ways, as Lorna (MSU) said in an interview, *'We're not meant to hold hands but I do hold hands with him.'*

I also found that if the rules were broken, expulsion from some placements of residency was often a result. Kate for example, had been sexually active at a previous unit, but was then moved to another unit. She was particularly distressed that *she* was the one who had to move. Kate clearly highlights in an interview that she would have liked a sexual relationship with her current boyfriend but their contact had been recently reduced due to the segregation:

Rebecca:	You can't have sexual intercourse here then?
Kate:	No we're not allowed, it's one of the hospital rules.
Rebecca:	What do you think about that?
Kate:	Well it would be alright if we were allowed at least once a month (laugh).
Rebecca:	do you have a boyfriend or . . . here?
Kate:	Yes, yes.
Rebecca:	Do you ever get to see him?
Kate:	No not at the minute because um, I used to see him all the time at the club you know before it got changed. Me and him were a bit cheesed off to tell you the truth.
Rebecca:	I can imagine.
Kate:	Because they're saying I'm vulnerable with men but what we did is we spoke to [staff] who runs the club, and we said to [staff], 'Has

there ever been a problem with us being sat together and talking and that?' and she said, 'No, but I'll have to admit this to you,' and I said, 'What?' She said 'I've been told to watch you especially,' and I said 'Why' and she said 'Because of your vulnerability.' So she says 'I've been keeping an eye on you over any of the other clients.'

Rebecca: And how do you feel about that?

Kate: It made me feel better actually knowing that she could truly say that there was nothing happening because she had been watching me, and knowing that if something had happened she would have reported it straight away and separated us. But I spoke to [psychiatrist] and I've asked him to make me go to mixed clubs because my fella's leaving in August and he's really upset, he were crying the other day because he can't see me often. And it upsets me to see him crying.

(Interview, client, LSU)

It is clear from these narratives that when women are perceived as specifically vulnerable, they invoke a need to be 'watched' and protected.

Kate's account shows that relationships on the wards can cause problems, in particular when people are due to move to other services or out into the community. In an interview with Louise, she suggested that certain relationships could cause problems for the day-to-day running of the wards, because she kept running away. When I asked her why she ran away and if it was to see her boyfriend, she replied saying, *'No. Because he upset me that much I didn't know how to cope with it.'* This shows that she wanted support, as Louise's repeated absconding was related to her relationship with her boyfriend at the time. Perhaps women were not requesting help and support because sexual relationships were prohibited and therefore dialogue on this subject was hindered. I would suggest that this issue is an illustration of the paternalism of services which has wide-reaching consequences.

Same sex relationships

Some of the clients had previously had sexual relationships with women. Despite the fact that there was a popular Lesbian, Gay, Bisexual and Transsexual (LGBT) support group and club at the unit, it seemed that more support and guidance for some of the women was needed. This is evidenced in my interview with Lorna when she told me that her girlfriend had just finished with her and that now she was going out with a man. She went onto say:

Lorna: It's complicated I know, staff find it complicated too.

Rebecca: Might you have a girlfriend in the future?

Lorna: No, I don't want another girlfriend, I've been there, done that, worn the tee-shirt and never going back. Staying with lads now. They're not as difficult, but saying that, they are.

Rebecca: So you had a girlfriend at your last hospital and one at this hospital but you've finished with girls now?

Lorna: Yes I won't have anything else to do with them.

Rebecca: Have you spoken to your therapist about this?

Lorna: Yes she's talked to me about it but she's said she's not the right person to deal with that so she'll transfer me to another therapist because she couldn't deal with the things that I was talking about.

(Interview, service user)

Lorna's experience illustrates the potential consequences of disclosing issues of a sexual nature; her bisexuality was treated as a specialist issue which required treatment by a particular therapist.

Andie told me that she was unsure about her sexuality, but her questioning was treated as disgusting by other clients as we can see here:

Andie: I didn't want to tell my friends in case I'm a freak, kind of way and that's why I didn't tell them last night I said 'I don't fancy lads.' A girl went 'Ew!' and I said 'What? It's nature. Different. Some lads are gay in here.'

Rebecca: Do you know there is a gay and lesbian (LGBT) club? Have you been offered to go to that?

Andie: I've been asked for it but staff here think it's not appropriate.

Rebecca: Not appropriate?

Andie: I'd like to go and talk to them and see what it's like being gay. It helps me because when I get out this hospital and go back to (home) and see a pretty girl. In my head I go 'Oh, she's pretty.' And I go up to her and go 'Wait a second, I need help and get some support' and go over and speak for the future, that's what I say.

Rebecca: Well perhaps you need some support with that, you need to talk to somebody about that. I mean why do you think the staff aren't letting you go?

Andie: Because I'm too young, because I'm only nineteen.

Rebecca: Yes but you're above the age of consent.

Andie: I'm 20 this year I think I'll be honest, I am gay, kind of thing but I do need some help with it.

(Interview, client, LSU)

In Andie's interview, a call for support was the main issue. Andie had been delayed from joining the LGBT group at the unit, which she was told was due to her being 'too young' but legally this was not the case.

Literature suggests that learning disabled women have little knowledge of same sex relationships due to the lack of information, role models and sex education, and some have very strong negative views about homosexuality (Burns and Davies, 2011; Hollomotz, 2011). Although my research shows that some women are interested in exploring their sexual identity, this was sometimes avoided by staff. This reflects staff attitudes similar to Yool et al.'s study which found that secure service staff did not think it was appropriate to discuss homosexuality with service users

(Yool et al., 2003). Staff members sometimes framed their concerns about gay relationships for the women as symptomatic of their past experiences, or again in terms of vulnerability, for example Adele a qualified staff member told me:

Adele: Some [women] have either chosen – not chosen to be gay – but decided that being gay is safer. That perhaps they weren't pre-disposed from an early age to be gay, but through circumstances have felt that it's safer to be with another woman and then there's others I think are just naturally and would have been gay no matter what . . . but then we get issues with vulnerability, like we've two women at the moment on the same ward who've been having a relationship, but one's more predatory than the other, so there's been a duty to keep the other one safe, so we've had to say 'no, you can't sit together', which sounds really punitive, but it's to keep one of them safe.

(Interview, qualified staff)

Some staff seemed to discuss clients and their sexuality using this 'predatory/ vulnerable' binary, possibly due to the common discourse around sexuality on the unit and its focus on risk. This has similarities with research focussing on teenage sexuality, for example Elliott (2010) who talks about the risks perceived by parents when their son or daughter embarks on a sexual relationship. The emphasis in these narratives about all client/client relationships on Unit C was that of protection from risk, and the problems that relationships can cause when one of the parties keeps getting hurt or manipulated. It was unclear whether staff were encouraging self-defence skills and healthy decision-making in the women or if it was simply controlling behaviour. Gwen Adshead recommends that secure service give more consideration to this issue:

> What is not explored sufficiently in forensic [secure] settings is the meaning of 'normal' sexual relationships for people who have experienced considerable childhood trauma and deprivation, and who are detained in long-term residential settings that are both custodial and therapeutic.
>
> (Adshead, 2004:83)

Two of the women in my study did not convey interest in sexual relationships, giving their negative past experiences as reasons. However, contrary to some research about learning disabled women (such as McCarthy, 1993; Fitzgerald and Withers, 2011), the remainder of the service user participants did want a sexual relationship. They wanted this despite the sexual abuse and violence in their pasts. In the face of the high levels of regulation they were subjected to, the women found a way to experience these intimate relationships in any way they could. As Carol Thomas explains, disabled people like all people, are both determined and determining (Thomas, 1999).

What is encouraging about my research is that women were managing to find ways to express themselves sexually, even though sexual relationships were regulated by the service. Individual staff 'allowed' some sexual expression in controlled ways (see also Christian et al., 2001), and policies and guidelines were individualised depending on risk factors. A reassuring point is that staff recognised the past experiences of the women as contributing to their challenging behaviour, rather than related to personality or impairments. A potential drawback to this, however, is that these experiences understandably elicit feelings of protection in staff, who become concerned about the balance between positive risk taking and protection.

I would argue again that this entrapment that women are experiencing is due to them being situated at the intersection of learning disability and gender, where issues of protection and paternalism proliferate (Björnsdóttir and Traustadóttir, 2010; Björnsdóttir et al., 2017). In addition to this are notions of female deviance, where offending is attributed to victimisation (Adshead, 2011). Ultimately, this can work against women's chances of resilience. Nevertheless, as Bernert points out:

> Equality and protection do not have to be an either/or priority if they are approached as an integrated process to enhance the sexual health and development of women with intellectual disabilities.
>
> (Bernert, 2011:140)

Conclusion

The relationships of women in my research were highly regulated. The concept of 'vulnerability' was a key part of this regulation, and from the stories about women which came out of the interviews, vulnerability was considered to be mainly a part of the woman, whether due to her impairment or history, rather than directly connected to the presence of male offenders at the unit. Stories of sexual violence and child abuse were very common with half of all interviewed clients disclosing such experiences, without being prompted. Some staff proposed that women have issues with repeating patterns of abuse, indicating that support and therapy should address this concern. Despite these experiences of abuse, and the potential problems of extra regulation related to the presence of male offenders, the majority of the women did not want to be segregated from the men socially.

Throughout this chapter, it becomes clear that the value and importance of relationships on Unit C is misrecognised. This is a phenomenon described in the literature as 'promoting independence' (Burns, 1993:104), and some authors claim concepts of independence proliferate because services are built on 'masculine' principles of self-sufficiency (Burns, 1993; Clements et al., 1995; Powell, 2001), whereas others suggest this is due to neoliberal policy making where premium is placed on individuals having freedom and choice (Hannah-Moffat, 2000; Kendall, 2004; Pollack and Kendall, 2005).

I would argue that all of these things come into play here. We have seen how the unit was set up mainly with men in mind, and how women staff had to argue for women-only spaces to be created. The discourse of predation and vulnerability, mainly due to the presence of men on the unit, instils feelings of protection and paternalism in staff, which in turn may encourage regulation of relationships between residents. The regulation of relationships appeared to be serving the interests of the organisation and staff rather than the residents (see also Grace et al., 2017) Also, the focus of 'independence' in policy for learning disabled people is a constant presence (Department of Health, 2001), as is the legacy of discourse surrounding institutionalised people, which presupposes people as at risk of relying on the institution (McWade, 2014) – these factors can result in positive relationships being treated with ambivalence.

One thing that was noticeable to me was the lack of family involvement in the service. Learning disabled people usually live with their families into adulthood, with their family providing their main system of support (Walmsley, 1996). Families generally know what is best for the person, what they respond to and what makes them more distressed. However, their involvement and consultation was not particularly evident here. I think the reason for this could be due to all the talk about negative family experiences and how it did not leave very much space for positive discussion. One of the staff roles seemed to be protecting clients from these negative relationships. When spending time with the clients, I became aware that even though they had experienced bad things at the hands of their family members, there was usually at least one person from their past with whom they retained a good relationship. It seems that efforts could be made to increase involvement and encourage positive links with families and friends.

Forcing clients who are experiencing different levels of distress to live together in close conditions may result in conflict and challenging behaviour, which can be described as effected by interpersonal influences (Clements et al., 1995). I did see evidence of frequent and intense conflict and aggression between clients, that superficially seemed to be about material items or family visits but was likely to reflect deeper issues. Clients described having their belongings damaged or stolen, as well as attacking and being attacked, physically and verbally, sometimes by name calling or threatening of family members. Issues of confidentiality sometimes provoked conflict, when clients considered other clients to be gossiping about them. A great deal of staff time was taken up by dealing with these conflicts, and finding ways to avoid contact between seemingly incompatible people.

Peer relationships were often not encouraged by staff or could even be discounted by them; staff might perceive them to be 'too personal', because of the issue of services promoting independence and autonomy. Staff can feel that 'they know best' about such relationships. This was not helpful and many clients would have liked their relationships to be encouraged and valued, even when one of the clients had moved on. My argument is that rather than constructing relationships as negative, it is possible to acknowledge difficulties and work towards supporting and encouraging them.

A key point in my argument is about staff/client relationships. Iona showed how a good therapeutic relationship can reduce or eliminate challenging behaviour, yet her behaviour was disapproved of by other staff who assumed she was giving the client special treatment. Powell (2001) advises that women who end up in secure care have a fundamental need for therapy and empowerment rather than containment and security, and claims that the treatment regime they are subjected to is based on a masculine model of secure services due to men being the majority group. This prevailing principle of masculinity is directly related to the expectation of independence.

Instead of promoting interdependence as I have recommended, I argue that the institution produces dependence. The next chapter looks at institutional practices examining how these maintain dependence and power imbalances, and indeed damage relationships.

Note

1 'No Longer a Diagnosis of Exclusion' (2003) is a Policy Implementation Guidance document published by the National Institute for Mental Health for England. This document states that therapy for people diagnosed as personality disordered should be well structured, have a clear focus and be coherent to both patient and therapist. Also, it should be relatively long-term, be well integrated with other services, and involve a clear treatment alliance between patient and therapist.

Bibliography

Adshead, G. (2004). More alike than different: Gender and forensic mental health. In N. Jeffcote & T. Watson (Eds.), *Working therapeutically with women in secure mental health settings* (pp. 78–90). London: Jessica Kingsley.

Adshead, G. (2011). Same but different: Constructions of female violence in forensic mental health. *International Journal of Feminist Approaches to Bioethics*, 4, 41–68.

Atkinson, D., Mccarthy, M., Walmsley, J., Cooper, M., Rolph, S., Aspis, S. . . . Ferris, G. (2000). *Good times, bad times: Women with learning difficulties telling their stories.* Kidderminster: BILD Publications.

Becker, D. (1997). *Through the looking glass: Women and borderline personality disorder.* Boulder, CO: Westview Press.

Bernert, D. J. (2011). Sexuality and disability in the lives of women with intellectual disabilities. *Sexuality and Disability*, 29, 129–141.

Björnsdóttir, K., Stefánsdóttir, Á., & Stefánsdóttir, G. V. (2017). People with intellectual disabilities negotiate autonomy, gender and sexuality. *Sexuality and Disability*, Early online version, 1–17.

Björnsdóttir, K., & Traustadóttir, R. (2010). Stuck in the land of disability? The intersection of learning difficulties, class, gender and religion. *Disability & Society*, 25, 49–62.

Bowlby, J. (2005). *A secure base: Clinical applications of attachment theory.* New York: Routledge.

Braye, S., Orr, D., & Preston-Shoot, M. (2010). *The governance of adult safeguarding: Findings from research into safeguarding adults boards.* Final report to the Department of Health. London: Department of Health.

Bressington, D., Stewart, B., Beer, D., & Macinnes, D. (2011). Levels of service user satisfaction in secure settings: A survey of the association between perceived social climate, perceived therapeutic relationship and satisfaction with forensic services. *International Journal of Nursing Studies*, 48, 1349–1356.

Burns, J. (1993). Invisible women-women who have learning disabilities. *The Psychologist*, 6, 102–104.

Burns, J., & Davies, D. (2011). Same-sex relationships and women with intellectual disabilities. *Journal of Applied Research in Intellectual Disabilities*, 24, 351–360.

Carnaby, S. (1998). Reflections on social integration for people with intellectual disability: Does interdependence have a role? *Journal of Intellectual and Developmental Disability*, 23, 219–228.

Christian, L., Stinson, J., & Dotson, L. A. (2001). Staff values regarding the sexual expression of women with developmental disabilities. *Sexuality and Disability*, 19, 283–291.

Clarkson, R., Murphy, G., Coldwell, J., & Dawson, D. (2009). What characteristics do service users with intellectual disability value in direct support staff within residential forensic services? *Journal of Intellectual and Developmental Disability*, 34, 283–289.

Clements, J., Clare, I., & Ezelle, L. (1995). Real men, real women, real lives? Gender issues in learning disabilities and challenging behaviour. *Disability & Society*, 10, 425–436.

Crawford, J. (2001). *The institutional hazard of being a visible woman*. The first International Conference on the care and treatment of learning disabled offenders. Preston: UCLAN.

Dein, K., & Williams, P. (2008). Relationships between residents in secure psychiatric units: Are safety and sensitivity really incompatible? *Psychiatric Bulletin*, 32, 284.

Department of Health. (2000). *No secrets: Guidance on developing and implementing multi-agency policies and procedures to protect vulnerable adults from abuse*. London: Department of Health.

Department of Health. (2001). *Valuing people: A new strategy for learning disability for the 21st century*. London: Department of Health.

Duperouzel, H. (2008). "It's OK for people to feel angry": The exemplary management of imminent aggression. *Journal of Intellectual Disabilities*, 12, 295–307.

Elliott, S. (2010). Parents' constructions of teen sexuality: Sex panics, contradictory discourses, and social inequality. *Symbolic Interaction*, 33, 191–212.

Fish, R. (2000). Working with people who harm themselves in a forensic learning disability service: Experiences of direct care staff. *Journal of Learning Disabilities*, 4, 193.

Fish, R., & Culshaw, E. (2005). The last resort? Staff and client perspectives on physical intervention. *Journal of Intellectual Disabilities*, 9, 93–107.

Fish, R., & Duperouzel, H. (2008). Just another day dealing with wounds: Self-injury and staff-client relationships. *Learning Disability Practice*, 11, 12–15.

Fitzgerald, C., & Withers, P. (2011). "I don't know what a proper woman means": What women with intellectual disabilities think about sex, sexuality and themselves. *British Journal of Learning Disabilities*, 41, 5–12.

Forchuk, C., Jewell, J., Schofield, R., Sircelj, M., & Valledor, T. (1998). From hospital to community: Bridging therapeutic relationships. *Journal of Psychiatric and Mental Health Nursing*, 5, 197–202.

Fulford, C., & Cobigo, V. (2016). Friendships and intimate relationships among people with intellectual disabilities: A thematic synthesis. *Journal of Applied Research in Intellectual Disabilities*. Available at http://onlinelibrary.wiley.com/doi/10.1111/jar.12312/full (Accessed 09/12/17).

Fyson, R., & Kitson, D. (2010). Human rights and social wrongs: Issues in safeguarding adults with learning disabilities. *Practice*, 22, 309–320.

Garland-Thomson, R. (2003). Integrating disability, transforming feminist theory. *NWSA Journal*, 14, 1–32.

Goffman, E. (1961). *Asylums: Essays on the social situation of mental patients and other inmates*. New York: Anchor Books, Doubleday & Co.

Goldberg, R. J., Higgins, E. L., Raskind, M. H., & Herman, K. L. (2003). Predictors of success in individuals with learning disabilities: A qualitative analysis of a 20-year longitudinal study. *Learning Disabilities Research & Practice*, 18, 222–236.

Goodwin, I. (1999). A qualitative analysis of the views of in-patient mental health service users. *Journal of Mental Health*, 8, 43–54.

Grace, N., Greenhill, B., & Withers, P. (2017). "They just said inappropriate contact": What do service users hear when staff talk about sex and relationships? *Journal of Applied Research in Intellectual Disabilities*. Available at http://onlinelibrary.wiley.com/doi/10.1111/jar.12373/full accessed 12/09/17

Hannah-Moffat, K. (2000). Prisons that empower. *British Journal of Criminology*, 40, 510–531.

Happell, B. (2008). Determining the effectiveness of mental health services from a consumer perspective: Part 1: Enhancing recovery. *International Journal of Mental Health Nursing*, 17, 116–122.

Harker-Longton, W., & Fish, R. (2002). "Cutting doesn't make you die": One woman's views on the treatment of her self-injurious behaviour. *Journal of Intellectual Disabilities*, 6, 137–151.

Herman, J. (1997). *Trauma and recovery: The aftermath of violence – from domestic abuse to political terror*. New York: Basic Books.

Hollomotz, A. (2011). *Learning difficulties and sexual vulnerability: A social approach*. London: Jessica Kingsley Publishers.

Hollomotz, A. (2013). Disability, oppression and violence: Towards a sociological explanation. *Sociology*, 47, 477–493.

Hornstein, G. A. (2013). Whose account matters? A challenge to feminist psychologists. *Feminism & Psychology*, 23, 29–40.

Hostick, T., & Mcclelland, F. (2002). "Partnership": A co-operative inquiry between community mental health nurses and their clients: 2: The nurse – client relationship. *Journal of Psychiatric and Mental Health Nursing*, 9, 111–117.

Howard, P. B., Clark, J. J., Rayens, M. K., Hines-Martin, V., Weaver, P., & Littrell, R. (2001). Consumer satisfaction with services in a regional psychiatric hospital: A collaborative research project in Kentucky. *Archives of Psychiatric Nursing*, 15, 10–23.

Kendall, K. (2004). Female offenders or alleged offenders with developmental disabilities: A critical overview. In W. R. Lindsay, J. L. Taylor & P. Sturmey (Eds.), *Offenders with developmental disabilities* (pp. 265–288). Oxford: Wiley.

Kittay, E. F. (2001). When caring is just and justice is caring: Justice and mental retardation. *Public Culture*, 13, 557–579.

Knox, M., & Bigby, C. (2007). Moving towards midlife care as negotiated family business: Accounts of people with intellectual disabilities and their families "just getting along with their lives together". *International Journal of Disability, Development and Education*, 54, 287–304.

Langley, G., & Klopper, H. (2005). Trust as a foundation for the therapeutic intervention for patients with borderline personality disorder. *Journal of Psychiatric and Mental Health Nursing*, 12, 23–32.

Lindsay, W. R., O'Brien, G., Carson, D., Holland, A. J., Taylor, J. L., Wheeler, J. R. . . . Johnston, S. (2010). Pathways into services for offenders with intellectual disabilities childhood experiences, diagnostic information, and offense variables. *Criminal Justice and Behavior*, 37, 678–694.

Linehan, M. M. (1993). *Skills training manual for treating borderline personality disorder*. New York: Guilford Press.

Lloyd, M. (2001). The politics of disability and feminism: Discord or synthesis? *Sociology*, 35, 715–728.

Markham, D. (2003). Attitudes towards patients with a diagnosis of "borderline personality disorder": Social rejection and dangerousness. *Journal of Mental Health*, 12, 595–612.

Markham, D., & Trower, P. (2003). The effects of the psychiatric label "borderline personality disorder" on nursing staff's perceptions and causal attributions for challenging behaviours. *British Journal of Clinical Psychology*, 42, 243–256.

Mccarthy, M. (1993). Sexual experiences of women with learning difficulties in long-stay hospitals. *Sexuality and Disability*, 11, 277–286.

Mccorkell, A. D. (2011). *Am I there yet? The views of people with learning disability on forensic community rehabilitation*. D.Clin.Psych. Thesis, University of Edinburgh.

Mcmillan, S., & Aiyegbusi, A. (2008). Crying out for care. In J. Clarke-Moore & A. Aiyegbusi (Eds.), *Therapeutic relationships with offenders: An introduction to the psychodynamics of forensic mental health nursing* (pp. 171–186). London: Jessica Kingsley.

Mcwade, B. (2014). *Recovery in an "arts for mental health" unit*. Ph.D. Thesis, Lancaster University.

Molvaer, J., Hantzi, A., & Papadatos, Y. (1992). Psychotic patients' attributions for mental illness*. *British Journal of Clinical Psychology*, 31, 210–212.

Morris, J. (1993). Feminism and disability. *Feminist Review*, 57–70.

Morrison, G. M., & Cosden, M. A. (1997). Risk, resilience, and adjustment of individuals with learning disabilities. *Learning Disability Quarterly*, 20(43), 43–60.

Murphy, G., Estien, D., & Clare, I. (1996). Services for people with mild intellectual disabilities and challenging behaviour: Service-user views. *Journal of Applied Research in Intellectual Disabilities*, 9, 256–283.

Nathan, R., Brown, A., Redhead, K., Holt, G., & Hill, J. (2007). Staff responses to the therapeutic environment: A prospective study comparing burnout among nurses working on male and female wards in a medium secure unit. *The Journal of Forensic Psychiatry & Psychology*, 18, 342–352.

National Institute for Mental Health in England. (2003). *Personality disorder: No longer a diagnosis of exclusion: Policy implementation guidance for the development of services for people with personality disorder*. London: Department of Health.

Nunkoosing, K., & John, M. (1997). Friendships, relationships and the management of rejection and loneliness by people with learning disabilities. *Journal of Intellectual Disabilities*, 1, 10–18.

Ogata, S. N., Silk, K. R., Goodrich, S., Lohr, N. E., Westen, D., & Hill, E. M. (1990). Childhood sexual and physical abuse in adult patients with borderline personality disorder. *American Journal of Psychiatry*, 147, 1008–1013.

Parrott, F. R. (2005). "It's not forever": The material culture of hope. *Journal of Material Culture*, 10, 245–262.

Parry-Crooke, G., & Stafford, P. (2009). *My life: In safe hands?* London: Metropolitan University.

Petersilia, J. (2000). Invisible victims: Violence against persons with developmental disabilities. *Human Rights*, 27, 9–12.

Pollack, S., & Kendall, K. (2005). Taming the shrew: Mental health policy with women in Canadian federal prisons. *Critical Criminology: An International Journal*, 13, 71–87.

Potier, M. A. (1993). Giving evidence: Women's lives in Ashworth maximum security psychiatric hospital. *Feminism & Psychology*, 3, 335–347.

Powell, J. (2001). Women in British special hospitals: A sociological approach. *Sincronia: Journal of Social Sciences and Humanities*, 5, 1–14.

Reed, J. (1994). *Report of the working party on high security and related psychiatric provision, volume 6.* London: Department of Health.

Reindal, S. M. (1999). Independence, dependence, interdependence: Some reflections on the subject and personal autonomy. *Disability & Society,* 14, 353–367.

Roffman, A. J. (2000). *Meeting the challenge of learning disabilities in adulthood.* Oxford: Brookes Publishing.

Rolph, S., Atkinson, D., Nind, M., Welshman, J., Brigham, L., Chapman, R. . . . Walmsley, J. (2006). Witnesses to change: Families, learning difficulties and history. *British Journal of Developmental Disabilities,* 52.

Sarkar, J., & Di Lustro, M. (2011). Evolution of secure services for women in England. *Advances in Psychiatric Treatment,* 17, 323–331.

Shattell, M. M., Andes, M., & Thomas, S. P. (2008). How patients and nurses experience the acute care psychiatric environment. *Nursing Inquiry,* 15, 242–250.

Shattell, M. M., Starr, S. S., & Thomas, S. P. (2007). "Take my hand, help me out": Mental health service recipients' experience of the therapeutic relationship. *International Journal of Mental Health Nursing,* 16, 274–284.

Stafford, P. (1999). *Defining gender issues: Redefining women's services.* London: WISH.

Thomas, C. (1993). De-constructing concepts of care. *Sociology,* 27, 649–669.

Thomas, C. (1999). *Female forms: Experiencing and understanding disability.* Buckingham: Open University Press.

Thomas, S., Shattell, M., & Martin, T. (2002). What's therapeutic about the therapeutic milieu? *Archives of Psychiatric Nursing,* 16, 99–107.

Thomson, M., & Johnson, P. (2017). Experiences of women with learning disabilities undergoing dialectical behaviour therapy in a secure service. *British Journal of Learning Disabilities,* 45, 106–113.

Tuffrey-Wijne, I., Bernal, J., Hubert, J., Butler, G., & Hollins, S. (2009). People with learning disabilities who have cancer: An ethnographic study. *British Journal of General Practice,* 59, 503–509.

Walmsley, J. (1993). Contradictions in caring: Reciprocity and interdependence. *Disability & Society,* 8, 129–141.

Walmsley, J. (1996). Doing what mum wants me to do: Looking at family relationships from the point of view of people with intellectual disabilities. *Journal of Applied Research in Intellectual Disabilities,* 9, 324–341.

White, G. W., Simpson, J. L., Gonda, C., Ravesloot, C., & Coble, Z. (2010). Moving from independence to interdependence: A conceptual model for better understanding community participation of centers for independent living consumers. *Journal of Disability Policy Studies,* 20, 233–240.

Wilkins, T., & Warner, S. (2001). Women in special hospitals: Understanding the presenting behaviour of women diagnosed with borderline personality disorder. *Journal of Psychiatric and Mental Health Nursing,* 8, 289–297.

Williams, V., & Robinson, C. (2001). "He will finish up caring for me": People with learning disabilities and mutual care. *British Journal of Learning Disabilities,* 29, 56–62.

Wolfson, P., Holloway, F., & Killaspy, H. (2009). *Enabling recovery for people with complex mental health needs: A template for rehabilitation services.* London: Faculty of Rehabilitation and Social Psychology, Royal College of Psychiatrists.

Wood, H., Thorpe, L., Read, S., Eastwood, A., & Lindley, M. (2008). Service user satisfaction in a low secure forensic learning disability unit? *Mental Health and Learning Disabilities Research and Practice,* 5, 176–191.

Yool, L., Langdon, P., & Garner, K. (2003). The attitudes of medium-secure unit staff toward the sexuality of adults with learning disabilities. *Sexuality and Disability*, 21, 137–150.

Portions of this chapter have been published as:

Fish, R. (2016). Friends and family: Relationships on the locked ward. *Disability and Society*, 31(10), 1385–1402. DOI: http://dx.doi.org/10.1080/09687599.2016.1261693

Fish, R. (2016). "They've said I'm vulnerable with men": Doing sexuality on locked wards. *Sexualities*, 19(5–6), 641–658. DOI: https://doi.org/10.1177/1363460715620574

5   Difficult women?[1]

The women at Unit C are dependent on the staff for many aspects of life: safety and reassurance, privileges and access to family, information about rules and notions of progression, as well as more practical things such as movement through spaces within the unit. This dependence allows the staff to exert control over the women's behaviours and influences the imbalance of power on the Unit. The power disparity is most salient when clients are subject to behavioural interventions. Much of the discourse about women when it comes to behavioural management, points to women as 'difficult' (Williams et al., 2001; Breeze and Repper, 1998), a reputation which precedes them, as I will show.

The assumption on Unit C is that women arrive at the unit in crisis or extreme distress, displaying behaviours that are considered to be in need of assessment and management. These behaviours may have been figured as causing the breakdown of their previous placement, or having been triggered by the move. Women are often placed in seclusion or on an 'observation level' as soon as they arrive, and staff say this is so they can assess the woman's needs. The aim, as expressed by qualified staff Adele, is to 'contain difficult behaviours' whilst supporting people to 'learn different ways of behaving in situations'. However, as Becker testifies, 'Surely, nothing distances [staff] so thoroughly from clients as the consideration of their "management" (Becker, 1997:140).

Special observations

At Unit C, clients who were deemed at risk of serious self-harm or suicidal behaviour, were put 'on a level', which meant they had to be watched at all times by staff. 'Level 3' or 'level 4' were the most extreme levels, meaning they had to be within eyesight or within arm's reach of staff at all times, respectively. However, both staff and clients pointed out that people were placed on a level *after* an incident of self-harm, which was too late. Dawn, a qualified staff had strong opinions about special observations:

Dawn: Special observation – I don't agree with it, I don't think it has a purpose. I think it does if people are suicidal. I think if people are suicidal at that point I think that it does have a purpose, because it has to be a short-term thing. I don't think it has a purpose within self-harm because people are generally put on them once they've self-harmed which is neither use nor ornament! Too late.

(Interview, qualified staff, LSU)

All of the women I spoke to pointed out that they did not like special observations. They felt that their privacy was being violated, feeling unable, for example, to go to the toilet when being watched:

Marion: I don't like it because they have to watch you having a bath and I don't like anybody seeing me undressed. I get embarrassed, I get really, really embarrassed and shown up. And they watch you when you go to the toilet and all that. I hate it, I really do! I feel like a murderer or something. I feel like they think I'm going to commit a crime.

(Interview, client, LSU)

Marion points out that this coercive strategy makes her feel subjected to custodial supervision as in a prison. Surveillance was being used here to make sure that clients behaved in a way staff wanted.

Barron (2002:76) demonstrates 'the close link between dependence (of assistance and support) and control' in her study of older learning disabled women who had moved out of institutions; she concludes that the women had been extensively subjected to others' views or criticisms about their behaviour from an early age. The motivation behind this critique had been to train and correct, resulting in the women adopting 'subservient positions', behaving as expected by staff and not challenging them. Yates suggests that this compliance arises because of the fundamental and tacit assumption of the service that staff are more able than service users, and thus are able to guide them and encourage 'valued' behaviours: 'Valued behaviours are commended; nonvalued behaviours, if not exactly punished, must be seen by the service user to be associated with undesired outcomes' (Yates, 2005:233). Yates describes how services use a range of tactics to do this, including record keeping, the inculcation of bodily disciplines, surveillance and more or less persuasive techniques for eliciting compliance.

As I have reported elsewhere, clients felt that they should be allowed to use self-harm if they needed to (Duperouzel and Fish, 2010) as they were not hurting anyone but themselves. Clients in this study agreed; Sarah, for example, told me she disliked being watched so much that it caused a further incident:

Sarah: I didn't like it. I really didn't like people watching me on the toilet, watching me get dressed. I just didn't like it, I said 'Get away from the door, I don't want you watching me', it put me off. I couldn't sleep because they were there, [I've] been on a level 4 as well and in your room. I can't sleep with them watching me. It puts me off sleeping, if someone's there watching you. [Even] on the toilet, I didn't like it. I said 'Get out of the room, I don't want you standing there' It put me off.

Rebecca: Did it make you more angry?

Sarah: Yes, then I trashed my room, chucked my TV and my digibox went with it, smashed it up. I said 'You're watching me' I said, 'You piss me off' so I went like that and I whizzed it and it broke. But I regretted it after because I had no telly to watch.

(Interview, client, MSU)

At times of distress, when women are placed on special observations, the intrusion of staff into their most private spaces makes them extremely angry; they will often harm themselves or damage their own precious items (Powell, 2001). Breaking important personal possessions seemed to be quite common in times of anger and frustration. Staff also felt uncomfortable about the use of special observations, yet the dilemma of whether to watch or to leave alone was not one that the support staff could make.

Monica points out here that engaging with the women at times like these can ensure that no further harm is done:

Monica: [Special observations] should be for as short a time as possible in response to a crisis and that's all. And they should be reduced back down as quickly. So if there's a crisis of self-harm, or if there's an attempted suicide or acute mental illness the support should be increased and then rapidly decreased, but sensibly decreased. And it should be used to engage with the client, not to sit with your feet up reading the paper and ignoring them. Because generally if they're on a high level of observation it's because they feel pretty crap, and then if you sit and you're mad that you're doing it, they're going to pick up on that and feel even crapper. And I've always said to people, 'If you're doing the one-to-one, you're with that person anyway, so why not play a board game, or if you're reading the paper read it with them. Do the crossword together, take them for a walk? If it's a woman, do her hair, if it's a man, even if you're sat watching footy, sit and watch it with him.' And use it to engage and talk to them because if they're going to talk and trust you they're likely to feel better quicker and be off the enhanced supervision. So that would be my gold standard.

(Interview, qualified staff, LSU)

Monica's views were supported by clients and most staff. When asked how the system should be changed, there was agreement between both groups that staff should use the time for being engaged with the woman and helping her to talk about her problems.

Rebecca: So if you have to be on a level and you understand why, because you might self-harm, what's the best way that staff can do it, what can they do to make it better for you?

Marion: Just to sit down together and listen to my problems.

(Interview, client, LSU)

There was, however, some debate about this engagement, as some people were worried that positive experiences of special observation may cause women to deliberately self-harm as a way of getting some one-to-one time with staff:

Adele: But the difficulty is that it's reinforcing, so you have to be really clear about the contingencies so you want to proactively offer. You want the client to ask for it. Once they ask for it they can get it in a proactive way before they've done something and that's when it works best, rather than getting it and feeling dependent on it.

(Interview, qualified staff)

In this excerpt, Adele picked up on the fact that special observations should be done proactively, and women should get to the point where they ask for enhanced support before self-harming. One member of staff told me that she was instructed not to engage with a secluded client, as it was considered to be 'reinforcing' – despite the client wanting to talk at this point. This point was confirmed by Adele's concerns about behavioural reinforcement.

The women had ideas about how being 'on a level' could be made less intrusive, and these were about staff bending the rules a little bit, for example just being there and not looking directly at the woman when she is on the toilet, or allowing the woman to go to the toilet in privacy:

Reenie: Um, well some staff, when I go to the toilet they will stand outside the door and just put their leg at the door, which I don't mind that. It's when they're standing at the toilet door with the door wide open [I don't like]. No, some staff close the door and just put their foot there and talk to me.

(Interview, client, LSU)

Annie: I get embarrassed with going to the bathroom, I don't like going to the bathroom in front of people. So they will say to me, if I'm unsettled then she says, 'No way,' she doesn't let me, but if I've been settled I'll say 'Look I want to go to the toilet, but give me two minutes and I'll be straight back out.' If I'm not out within that two minutes she comes in. If I've done something I've got no leg to stand on I can't argue the toss because I've betrayed that trust.

(Interview, client, LSU)

Reenie pointed out that staff can interpret the policy flexibly and in different ways, some are able to be more discreet than others. Annie equated this flexibility with 'trust', in that the staff member was bending the rules but expecting that Annie would not expose this by self-harming. As seen in the previous chapter, trust is an important dimension of the staff/client relationship and works two ways. Being trusted can result in flexibility of rules; however, there are consequences. If someone is trusted, then there are expectations about their behaviour, and if trust is broken, this can turn into blame, as Jackie described here:

Jackie: So it's such an interesting issue, special observations, and I can completely see why the staff get resentful sitting outside somebody's room
and doing that for ages and watching them on the toilet, and women
getting really cross and losing their privacy and their dignity, and [staff
think] 'Well if you weren't doing this then we wouldn't have to be doing
this.' And then it gets a bit of a punitive aspect to it.

(Interview, qualified staff)

It is evident from Jackie's reflection that the expectation is for clients to 'self-direct' as Goffman (1961) observed, and the use of observation is the way of driving this. Furthermore, the use of observation may be blamed on the client, as though it is a natural consequence of failing to self-direct. Special observation is extremely relevant to all relationships on the locked ward. It can be an opportunity for improving or even damaging the staff/client relationship, and it can cause problems with other clients. Self-harm still happens when observation is not being employed, and sometimes when it is. Therefore, the ongoing and frequent use of observation in this setting is not achieving its goal. Engagement, however, is reported to be more effective and a realistic alternative to the feelings of dehumanisation caused by constant observation (Bowles et al., 2002; Cutcliffe and Barker, 2002). I suggest that effectual engagement, described as such in policy, and most importantly implemented in practice, is a more appropriate and progressive model than observation. Engagement in the form of staff/client relationships is credited as reducing incidents of self-harm, where the traditional response has been prevention using special observation, as well as confiscation of belongings which could be used for harm.

Removal of belongings

Clients were often subjected to the removal of their belongings because of their self-harm and this caused difficulties in therapeutic relationships. In my previous research with learning disabled women in a similar service, I found that self-harm can put a strain on the staff/client relationship because of a conflict of interests; staff were trying to prevent self-harm in order to protect clients' well-being, yet clients felt the need to use the behaviour as a coping strategy in times of stress (Fish and Duperouzel, 2008). Further, staff were feeling blamed by management when clients had self-harmed which caused emotions such as anger and betrayal.

Women in my study reported that self-harm was very important to them as a coping strategy. Aiyegbusi proposes that women who self-harm experience their bodies as 'detached' and use them to express the 'non-verbal narrative of their traumatic history' (Aiyegbusi, 2002:143). In this sense, acts of self-harm represent a bodily narrative to enact distress. Self-harm is described by women as a 'release' from mental pain and as a way of communicating this pain (Harker-Longton and

Fish, 2002). All except one of the women clients I spoke to told me that they had self-harmed at some point in their lives. Most had started before the age of 10, in response to a distressing situation such as abuse or a death or conflict within their family. The women who still self-harmed told me that arguments on the ward or being apart from their family were the causes for their current self-harm, for example:

Rebecca:	When did you start self-harming?
Lorna:	Age seven.
Rebecca:	Age seven! Can you remember it?
Lorna:	Yes.
Rebecca:	Why did you do it?
Lorna:	Because I'd had an argument with my mum so I cut all my legs.
Rebecca:	And you've carried on ever since?
Lorna:	Yes, started with my arms though.
Rebecca:	What do you feel like when you self-harm?
Lorna:	I feel sad when I self-harm so I do it to get the release out, I don't feel better after it, I still feel sad, but it's kind of got a little bit out, not much though.
Rebecca:	Are they helping you on here to think of different ways to get the release?
Lorna:	They're trying to help me, yes. They try and they give you all the support they can, but there's only a certain amount of support they can give me, and I'm just not willing to [stop], I am, but I'm not, if you know what I mean?
Rebecca:	Can you see yourself stopping self-harming?
Lorna:	With help yes.
Rebecca:	Is there anything that helps you?
Lorna:	Talking to staff sometimes, but not always.
Rebecca:	What kind of things make you want to self-harm?
Lorna:	I have arguments with other clients, um, when I spoke to my ex-partner, things like that. My little brother, because I miss him.
Rebecca:	Why do you think you do it?
Lorna:	Just to say to people how upset I am and for myself.

(Interview, client, MSU)

Lorna spoke openly about the reasons and functions of her self-harm, in particular the 'release' from distress that it offered her and the materialisation of this distress which she said can be caused by arguments with other clients. Conflicts between clients were often mentioned as reasons for self-harm, as well as worrying about family. Prior to my previous research into self-harm, organisations such as Unit C had a policy of prevention, to try to stop self-harming altogether, which caused many issues including staff feeling blamed when someone self-harmed. Now, Unit C has a 'harm minimisation' policy, implemented in response to research findings. This policy allows staff to recognise that self-harm is a coping strategy used by some people and places the responsibility for their behaviour onto the client. Some clients, after risk assessment, are 'allowed' to self-harm whilst they work through the reasons and try to find alternative coping strategies. Other clients, who are deemed to want to self-harm in a riskier way, are excluded from this system. The tools staff use to prevent self-harm for these clients include removing belongings from the person, special observation and physical intervention. All of the women recognised why these measures were being used, but reported that they were not happy at the time of implementation. Marion, for example had all her CDs taken out of her room to prevent her from using them to harm herself:

Rebecca: Do you mind when they take [your belongings] away?
Marion: Well no, well I do, I get upset about them but then I realise they're doing it for the best, trying to help me, because they don't want to see me in pain, they don't want to see me hurt. It's part of their job to look after us patients and do it well.

(Interview, client, LSU)

Marion recognised that one of the roles of staff was to 'look after' the women, and she saw the removal of her belongings as a sign of this protection. Certainly, removal of belongings was used on Unit C to manage clients, as an approach to prevent incidents of self-harm, and this often worked because great importance was placed on personal possessions. This was particularly relevant with CDs and music, as women used their music as a way to relax in their room and used musical preferences as part of their identity. Being dispossessed was construed as punishment.

There is research about reasons for and functions of self-harm in secure learning disability services, including work I was involved in (Liebling et al., 1997; James and Warner, 2005; Duperouzel and Fish, 2008; Fish and Duperouzel, 2008; Duperouzel and Fish, 2010) which has informed policy and NHS NICE guidance (National Institute for Health and Care Excellence, 2011). Some research incorporates relationships into the discussions, for example Smith and Power (2014) report that self-harm in both men and women begins at an early age and is in response to some sort of abuse. They found that women who had managed to stop self-harming invoked relationships as their main motivation, highlighting the role of verbalisation, social engagement and openness to therapy as a conduit to recovery. Many of the women I spoke to pointed out that having someone to talk to might stop them wanting to self-harm, and that having time to talk to staff helped them to feel better. For example:

Rebecca: What happens after you've banged your head? Do you feel a bit better?
Ellie: Yeah. I calm down then and then I talk to staff
Rebecca: And do you want to be able to not do it in the future?
Ellie: Uh huh. Yeah.
Rebecca: If you're thinking about scary things from the past, is there anything that can help you not to bang your head?

Ellie:	On Friday, [staff] got a file and we were looking at the bars saying the different colours and what mood it makes you and that and how I feel in seclusion and that.
Rebecca:	And was that okay?
Ellie:	Yeah. I've done that and we carried on and we started talking about other things.
Rebecca:	Okay. So basically having somebody to talk to can help you?
Ellie:	Yeah.

(Interview, client, LSU)

Ellie pointed out that therapeutic activities with staff helped her to think through and talk about her feelings. This was a theme throughout the discussions about self-harm, in particular when women had returned from difficult therapy sessions, time to talk with staff was important to them and therapeutic (see also Parry-Crooke and Stafford, 2009), and conversely, if staff were not available to talk, the woman may feel like self-harming, as I show in my fieldnotes here:

Jane is in the living room and she is crying. I ask her what is wrong and she tells me that she is in pain because she has swallowed batteries from her TV remote and nobody is helping her. She thinks they are stuck. A male member of staff comes into the room and says there is nothing he can do, batteries will cause pain if swallowed and Sarah will just have to wait for them to pass through her body. He offers her some Senna to help them pass, and a magnetic scan to check where they are. I ask her why she did it, and she tells me that her therapy session this morning was very upsetting and when she came back to the ward there was nobody to talk to about it.

(Fieldnotes, MSU)

Rather than planning for such events, and allowing staff to put time aside for engagement after therapy, the organisational response to self-harm was to put formal special observation methods in place as I have described.

Aggression

Physical aggression, in the form of aggression by women towards other clients and staff members was common on the ward. Concepts of aggression were very much influenced by the gender of the clients in Unit C. In some ways, the women were defined by their style of aggression: forms of conflict considered to be masculine were valued over those regarded as feminine. Three staff articulated the commonly held beliefs:

John:	The lads would tend to come up to you, hit you once, then back off, whereas the women would be more low level, 'tapping' at you constantly.

(Interview, unqualified staff)

Stewart: Typically, the lads are – I'm trying to think of an okay word – you still
need your boundaries with the blokes, but they're more reserved in
their planning and things like that . . . They could still be devious for
want of a better word, but they wouldn't be, usually, as emotive as
when you're working with the women really.

(Interview, qualified staff)

Wendy: It's a different area, working with the women, they're very – more
demanding than what the men would be. The men would probably
shout and scream and get it over in one go where the women would go
on for days at a time.

(Interview, unqualified staff)

Descriptions of women's aggression as low level, prolonged and persistent were
common. Women were described as more devious, manipulative, drawing out
their conflicts for longer than necessary. 'Feminine' styles of aggression were
given as explanations for the greater use of coercive measures with women, as
evidenced by this quote:

Adele: I know it's a sweeping generalisation – but I think men are a little bit
easier to understand in that you can say, 'He gets very angry about this,
and he'll hit someone and be aggressive for half an hour', and it's more
predictable, whereas I think with women they can maybe keep an incident going for days. It can be verbal aggression, then leading to threats,
then leading to hostility, then an actual assault or self-harm, or some act
that leads to seclusion or whatever and it can carry on. And I think staff
get frustrated, desperate, burnt out. And I don't think it's intentional
and I don't think it's 'Oh, she's a woman so we'll seclude her', I don't
think it's that. I think staff get a bit desperate with women.

(Female qualified staff)

Adele acknowledged that she was making a generalisation, but her words show
how staff respond to the type of aggression shown by the women. The concept
that women 'burn out' staff is a common one that I have heard often during my
years of research. 'Relational' aggression indicates the use of relational factors to
bring harm or cause upset to someone and generally features in literature about
children and adolescents (Crick and Grotpeter, 1995; Cullerton-Sen et al., 2008),
indicating its socially constituted nature. Relational aggression (as compared to
overt aggression) is said to be more subtle and covert and more likely to be a cause
of stress among staff due to emotional exhaustion (Oddie and Ousley, 2007). In
line with this, staff at Unit C often considered women's aggression in terms of
their past experiences, and the means they have used to survive them:

Iona: When I started to think about how she behaved, I put it in context of
a very abusive past and a very, very abusive present. Then I started to

understand it, then I started to think about all the other women I've cared for and why they behave the way that they do, because a lot of the women do behave in a very extremely emotionally charged way either by manipulation or by screaming or shouting or by aggression. A lot of it was very, it put women in context for me, even if they don't openly say they've had an abusive past I could see, you sort of patch it all together.

(Interview, qualified staff)

Women's violence was often looked at in terms of their pasts on Unit C, including the use of attachment theory (Bowlby, 1977) as I have shown in the previous chapter. Encouragingly, as I have described, attachment theory was used by some staff to explain why some clients were aggressive with them when they were finishing a shift, for example, and as described, women were talked about as behaving in a way which fulfilled their needs in the past but which is considered maladaptive in current situations. Certainly, there were attempts to help women to see the effects of their actions in community meetings (explained in Chapter 4), so pasts were not always considered to be permanently damaging. In the next chapter, I argue that past experiences can be kept in mind whilst working towards the future, and therefore these two concerns are not mutually exclusive.

Women who live in learning disability services are subjected to predetermined views on the way their aggression is conceived. Their aggression may be attributed to their cognitive ability, frustration with communication skills, or as a challenge to ward rules and this demarcation can result in differing attributions and treatment (Secker et al., 2004; Wilcox et al., 2006; Kleinberg and Scior, 2014).

Consequently, learning disabled women's aggression is often described as 'challenging behaviour' (Clements et al., 1995), the most popular definition of which is:

abnormal behaviour(s) of such intensity, frequency or duration that the physical safety of the person or others is placed in serious jeopardy, or behaviour which is likely to seriously limit or deny access to the use of ordinary community facilities.

(Emerson, 2001:3)

This label is generally used for learning disabled people, children with learning difficulties or those with dementia and has been criticised in the literature as locating the responsibility within the individual, and overshadowing other issues such as deficient support (Mason and Scior, 2004; Chan, 2012).

The use of the word 'challenge' implies some sort of power struggle, which has led some researchers to suggest that the terminology may influence staff perceptions and responses to the behaviour (Chan, 2012). The word 'challenge' was used on Unit C to describe women's behaviour; for example Adele discussed the connection between behaviour and incarceration:

Adele: Obviously everybody that is here is here because their behaviour challenges society in one way or another. Now that may be that it challenges society in terms of forensic offending and they've actually been through the court process. It may be that it challenges society in terms of self-harm for instance, that services in the community can't cope with and that they are considered to be such a degree of danger to themselves or others that they need separating from society for a brief period of time to learn more appropriate behaviour.

(Interview, qualified staff)

All of this information is pointing to women's violence and aggression as the problem of the individual, whether down to their gender, impairment or past experiences, or a combination of the three. Context is not being given due credit, in contrast, as Kendall points out, 'challenging behaviour, however potentially threatening, can be viewed as purposeful once it is contextualised' (Kendall, 2004:273). If effective staff/client relationships can reduce levels of violence as I argued in Chapter 4, this suggests that many incidents do relate to context and ward environment.

We have seen how aggression is conceptualised at Unit C, as having particular manifestations in women and as a response to past trauma. Considering this, how effective are the tools and strategies used to deal with aggression and violence on the wards?

Physical intervention

Physical intervention or restraint is used to restrict someone's freedom of movement when there is the threat of injury to others or damage to property. Specialist staff at Unit C have developed a distinct system of physical intervention (and related training for staff) that involves different levels of intervention (breakaway, physical intervention and enhanced physical intervention). The body of literature about physical intervention and its use in learning disability services is very small. Sequeira and Halstead (2001) found that the use of physical intervention could cause pain and be construed as punishment, and participants in Fish and Culshaw's (2005) study described feeling retraumatised by the episode of restraint; in that being overpowered by another person reminded them of violence and abuse in their pasts. Not all women in the current study had experienced being physically restrained, and the ones who hadn't were very quick to point this out, demonstrating the stigma involved. Those who had not recently experienced restraint, equally told me how long it had been since their last incident. Women did not like being restrained, particularly when other people were watching:

Kate: It made me feel awful because when I was restrained my top come up a little bit, OK it was only my belly showing but that's bad enough. I'm a woman, I was being restrained by three men. Yes, there was two women and three men. And there was other men in the room making sure that I didn't attack anyone whilst being restrained.

(Interview, client, LSU)

Most of the women who had been restrained reported that it felt painful. Worryingly, it seems that the women were not given specific instructions about when restraint would be used. Helen, a client, told me in an interview: *'They don't tell you they're going to restrain you, you just know that if you do an act they're going to respond in that way.'* This statement implies that there is no warning prior to restraint, or guidance in place that the women have been made aware of. When asked how this arrangement could be improved, the women requested that staff talk to them and ask what is bothering them, possibly going with them to another room, for example:

Brenda: Talking. Talking to us more . . . Talking to us more seeing why we're angry, letting us try to explain who we're angry with.
Rebecca: Yeah, so you could get it out before?
Brenda: Yeah, let us try to explain.

(Interview, client, MSU)

If restraint has to be used, all of the women suggested that staff should be engaged with the client at all times:

Rebecca: Is it better if they're talking to you all the time?
Bonnie: Yes, not giving me no contact makes me worse. If they're holding me but not talking to me, I'm trying to talk to them and they don't talk to you back, that really does my head in and I go worse.

(Interview, client, LSU)

Talking with staff was important to all the women, and some said that humour was a good way to calm them down. Humour is sometimes used as a way to de-escalate a situation before restraint is used; however, Ellie pointed out that staff laughing during restraint is hurtful:

Rebecca: What about talking to you [during restraint]? Do you like it?
Ellie: Yeah, but not having a laugh and that when you've been unsettled.
Rebecca: No.
Ellie: Just sit there and talk about what's upsetting me, which I prefer that.
Rebecca: Yeah, okay. And what about when you're in restraint do they say how long you're going to be in it and why?
Ellie: They say 'are you calming down?' And if I'm calm they let go, but if I'm not settling down it's harder. They ask me if I'd take PRN [as required medication] and if I say no and then they ask me again, and sometimes it leads to seclusion and sometimes I take the PRN.

(Interview, client, LSU)

Ellie pointed out that staff offer her a PRN if she is unsettled, which is usually taken in pill form but in cases of extreme distress can be forcibly given as an injection. I did see women requesting PRNs on the wards and being offered them, before the need for restraint as Adele suggested earlier when talking about special observation. Some research studies argue that the use of PRN as a proactive method is preferable to women than more coercive methods (e.g. Veltkamp et al., 2008). Ellie also said that she does not appreciate staff using humour in this situation. The use of humour for de-escalating aggression is discussed in the literature as effective on occasion (Duperouzel, 2008), but it clearly is best used only by knowledgeable staff who have built up a relationship with the client, as Adele suggested here:

Adele: It's about knowing your person again. There are some people for whom humour works and you can de-escalate a situation very quickly with humour. There are some people for humour is the big trigger and you wouldn't go there and you wouldn't make a joke of the situation, so it's about knowing the person that you're working with. In some instances, you could remind them of positive things that are going to happen later on, and that's enough to make them stop and think about, 'Oh I don't really want to do this because I don't want to not be able to do that thing,' and equally just reminding somebody of something may be the trigger to further escalation. So it really does come down to knowing the person to be perfectly honest. Which I think is so hard for people like bank staff[2] to know, and I'm sure that there are more incidents that happen with unfamiliar staff than with familiar staff.

(Interview, qualified staff)

Adele's comment makes an argument for the importance of the therapeutic relationship; the better the therapeutic relationship is, the more the staff member knows how to work with the client. The importance of staff/client relationships in terms of knowing what works with individual clients was discussed in Chapter 4, and it is crucial to consider the impact of power imbalances on these relationship when living in such close confinement. Adele's comment demonstrates this when she points out that humour may curtail a situation for some people but not others, and the same goes for using incentives for good behaviour. Supportive relationships are very important for clients' progression, and they also seem to contribute to behavioural stability. According to Herman's concept of recovery (Herman, 1997), the growth of the therapeutic relationship can protect against the perceptions of repetition of past traumas as described so often in the literature about coercive methods (e.g. Aitken and Noble, 2001). Herman explains it as: '(a) shared understanding of the survivor's characteristic disturbances of relationship and the consequent risk of repeated victimization offers the best insurance against unwitting re-enactments of the original trauma in the therapeutic relationship' (Herman, 1997:127). Attachment theory, as I described earlier, also recommends building stable attachments as 'springboards' to positive future relationships (Bowlby, 2005). Relationships therefore are central to my argument. Evidently, incidents of aggression and self-harm along with the corresponding use of coercive methods are reduced when staff/client relationships are at their best. Unfortunately, however, some opportunities to strengthen staff/client relationships on Unit C were being wasted.

As with special observation and other coercive methods, there were concerns that clients would engineer incidents of restraint so that staff engage with them; therefore sometimes staff were told not to interact with clients during such situations, for example:

Karen: That's another thing, sometimes, sometimes the guidelines are not to interact with them because they want that interaction and they want that touch. Some of them it's a sexual thing, and some want other women to be holding them all the time and talking to them. So then the guidelines say there's no interaction, make it quite boring for them, make it that it's not a good experience, in the fact that it's boring and it's not stimulating. Others that are very, very damaged, you would talk and just say things like you know, 'We're here, talk to us, you're safe' that kind of stuff. So it's all individual.

(Interview, qualified staff)

Karen making the point that clients may be *engineering* aggression in order to gain some sort of engagement suggests that clients are not receiving the responsiveness they need, or conversely that their anger is not considered legitimate and the context is denied. Another concerning matter was that there was no debrief after incidents of restraint. It could be argued that for staff and clients to learn from the situation at hand, it would be beneficial for them to discuss it afterwards and tell each other how they felt, as Jackie suggested here:

Jackie: Well it's surreal, I've always thought that if you were watching some of the things that happen on some of the flats here you would think 'what on earth is happening? How does that work that this restraint happens and then there isn't – not reconciliation – but there isn't a process that goes after? You don't want to reinforce something by having a physical intervention and then having a big confab or something, but some forum where you enable staff and clients to be able to talk with each other in an open and honest way, so that the staff aren't there as objects, or aren't seen as staff: 'They don't necessarily have feelings. They're there to do their job, they're there to sort this out and we are on the receiving end of this, But that makes us really angry, that we are.' We need to acknowledge some of that stuff and share the responsibility because it's 'You made me feel like this,' and, 'You did that.' So if you don't discuss it – to me communication's everything – it's an openness.

(Interview, qualified staff)

Jackie's point about how life might look to an outsider indicates how conflict and resolution on the wards is very different from the outside world. Jackie was pointing to debriefing as a way of developing understanding between staff and clients, a way for everyone to understand how these situations make people feel. Yet, her comment still reflects the dominant discourse of behavioural reinforcement. She went on to explore the whole concept of using coercive methods with the women:

> *Jackie:*   I'm really conflicted about it if I'm being honest, because I just think that, on the one hand I think these methods are probably necessary, on the other hand I just think once they happen it's like a line gets crossed and it confirms something to the individual woman client, that you wouldn't want to have them confirm to themselves. Like 'I'm so bad and out of control that I have to have this happen to me.'
>
> *(Interview, qualified staff)*

Jackie's concept of 'a line getting crossed' is one I have heard a number of times. Staff worry that these coercive methods are self-fulfilling due to their routine use, that the women will see these methods being used and accept that they are needed, and that this creates a downward spiral of events. I maintain that therapeutic relationships are the only way to stop the spiral and create new possibilities; the importance of relationships continues throughout these themes. If staff know clients well, they are aware of their characteristics and how to be together in the safest possible way; and it could be argued that encouraging this accommodation is key to implementing the social model of disability. Good relationships can bring about 'behavioural stability', and undeniably are key to clients' progression throughout services.

Seclusion

Aggression is described as extremely damaging to the staff/client relationship; however, if the threat of aggression continues and physical intervention is deemed to have gone on for too long, the service advocates the use of seclusion.

Seclusion is used on Unit C when clients become unmanageably aggressive and physical intervention is not containing their behaviour. The Mental Health Act Code of Practice defines the practice of seclusion as *'the supervised confinement of a patient in a room, which may be locked. Its sole aim is to contain severely disturbed behaviour which is likely to cause harm to others.'* The document goes on to advise that:

> *Seclusion should be used only as a last resort and for the shortest possible time. Seclusion should not be used as a punishment or a threat, or because of a shortage of staff. It should not form part of a treatment programme.*
>
> (Department of Health, 2007:122–123)

Seclusion continues to be a commonly used intervention in psychiatric services (Hoekstra et al., 2004) and in learning disability services (Emerson, 2001). A controversial form of containment, seclusion is often considered by service users to be punitive, obstructive in the development of therapeutic relationships (see Gilburt et al., 2008) and even a violation of human rights (McSherry, 2017).

Research literature that includes service users' experiences of seclusion often reports that they are confused about the reasons for being secluded, which causes fear and trepidation (e.g. Brown and Tooke, 1992). This seemed to be the case in Unit C, with one service user pointing out that she was secluded for swearing:

Rebecca: Do you ever have to go to the seclusion room?

Kate: No, I did when I first come in but that member of staff who put me in there got told off by the doctor for putting me in there because all I did was tell him to fuck off. Because he were trying to calm me down and I weren't interested because I'd been bullied at the club. I weren't interested so I told him to fuck off and leave me alone. That's all I did, I didn't try to strike him I didn't do nothing I just said 'Fuck off [name] I don't want to know.' So when my doctor came to let me out she said 'You shouldn't have put her in there for doing that.'

Rebecca: And so at that point you didn't realise why you were being secluded?

Kate: No, I was really scared I actually peed myself through being frightened. I wet myself!

(Interview, client, LSU)

It seems that Kate was not made aware of why she was secluded, or involved in any debriefing afterwards. She also pointed out how afraid the experience made her feel.

It seems that services sometimes use seclusion to remove a person from a situation of conflict, even when they are not the aggressor. Here, another service user described being secluded for reasons other than her own aggression:

Rebecca: Why did you get secluded?

Andie: Because [another client] she'd been whacking me all night, calling my family names. I got angry with her, my first time when I came, I didn't do nothing to her. I was nervous, upset, I went to seclusion room with [two staff members]. They both put me in there in there, behind this wall and I'd been sleeping in there, I sleep in there for a bit, not all night. I had to have a tissue on my head, it had been bleeding a bit.

(Interview, client, LSU)

A staff member, John, also explained that the reasons for seclusion are not always clear. Here he suggested that clients were sometimes secluded for the sake of others who live on the flats:

John: I don't like the layout of the seclusion rooms, I think it damages [clients] more. But a lot of the time you've got to bring [name] out of the flat because she's disrupting all the others.

Rebecca: Do you think it would be better to have some kind of high dependency suite rather than seclusion?

John: I think that would be better. A lot of the time at night they put [name] in at night, a lot, because all the other girls are in bed and she's in seclusion and she probably doesn't need to be in, but they've got to get her out of the flat for the sake of the other girls.

(Interview, support worker, LSU)

John suggested that it was not aggression that was the cause for seclusion, but 'disruption' – the seclusion room was being used for another purpose here. Another staff member was more specific about reasons for seclusion:

Rebecca: Why do you put somebody into seclusion, what would be the reason?
Karen: Just heightened, yes aggression and you've been restraining for over 40 minutes and you would put them in.

(Interview, qualified staff, MSU)

Because of the guidance and time limits for using physical restraint, if somebody is not calming down after being restrained for a certain period of time, staff decide to use seclusion as a method to 'calm the person down', or even just to end the restraint. However, many service users in the literature point out that being placed in seclusion makes them feel more angry (e.g. Chamberlin, 1985) because of the feelings of powerlessness it evokes. Here, Sarah described feeling angrier when in seclusion:

Rebecca: Is high dependency similar to seclusion?
Sarah: No in seclusion, you do four hours in there and if you still don't calm you down they can put you in for another four hours, because I stayed in there for eight hours because I didn't calm down. I banged my head and had a big lump out here, kept banging and banging.
Rebecca: Why were you banging your head?
Sarah: Stressed. I always do it, go in seclusion I just smash my head. I had a piece of string in my pocket, they got my pocket and they didn't get everything out and I got the string and cut myself in seclusion.
Rebecca: When you think about that, what do you feel like, why did you cut yourself?
Sarah: Because I was angry.

(Interview, client, MSU)

The decision to place someone in seclusion should be a last resort measure when somebody has become so angry that it impossible to reason with them; however, it seems that when the decision is made, the person is no longer consulted or engaged with by staff. This means that the issue which caused the anger may not be dealt with or resolved, and relationships might be put at risk. Also, clients not being aware of the criteria for seclusion highlights the power imbalance inherent in the staff/client relationship as staff are in control of this eventuality. All of these issues demonstrate the damage that these coercive methods can do to relationships.

The seclusion room environment

I did not witness any incidents of physical intervention or seclusion during my fieldwork, possibly because I was a new and 'interesting' presence on the ward, and I did not spend enough time on each ward to become familiar enough to people. When I was on the wards, clients often wanted to talk to me rather than other staff or clients, which may have provided a distraction from contentious issues. I did, however, see women who were already in seclusion, through the window and I was shown the seclusion rooms in both areas:

> The seclusion suite in the LSU has a door leading from each flat, a toilet room, and a door leading into the seclusion room. There is a 2ft by 1ft window in the door and conical mirrors at the back of the room in the corners which work to show the observer areas not visible from this window. A staff member is required to observe at all times. The only furniture is a bed, which is moulded in with the floor and holds a wipe-clean mattress. Lights and sprinkler on the ceiling are covered with rounded plastic.
>
> (Fieldnotes, LSU)

Many of the participants in my research talked about the physical aspects of the seclusion room. Here, a staff member discussed the logistics of seclusion, and how difficult it is to seclude a person:

Dawn: You lay them face down on the bed and put their arms behind them like that and somebody holds them. And then you have somebody kneeling on their legs and their legs are up as well. So you have everybody gets off, and the last person is there and that person, what you're supposed to do is have two people holding and one kneeling on their legs while their legs, and drag that person out of the room. Well our bed's there and our door's there, so if that person's on the bed, you're not dragging them in a straight line for one, and also as you're trying to move the mattress moves off the bed. So it works but it's very difficult.

(Interview, qualified staff, LSU)

From this description it is easy to imagine how difficult it would be to maintain someone's dignity when moving them to the seclusion room. The process of moving a person to this room sounds extremely unpleasant and would clearly attract a lot of attention from anyone in the surrounding area. Some of the women commented on the visibility of this procedure.

Furthermore, some of the women pointed out that the room was too cold, and others commented that the room was uncomfortable:

Rebecca: So what did it feel like when you were in seclusion?
Kate: It were awful because it's bare walls there's nothing in there. Nothing in there, they even took the mattress off me because some clients will put the mattress against the door so you can't see in. And they didn't want me doing that so they took the mattress. So I sat on a wooden bench, basically it's harder than [wood] because it's reinforced.

(Interview, client, LSU)

If the surroundings are uncomfortable and the door is locked, seclusion may be construed as punishment (Phillips, 2005); this may also be an issue when people feel as though others can see them in the seclusion room. There were many issues about the lack of privacy when secluded:

Kate: When someone's in seclusion, and we have to get on the front desk or something we can see whoever's in seclusion because we're going through there, and we can see whoever's in seclusion. So it's not fair on that person who's in seclusion. Like they used to put, when someone were walking past we used to say to them 'We're coming through, can you safeguard that person?' So they used to put a black binbag up for a couple of seconds against the window so you couldn't see who it were, but they don't do that any more.

(Interview, client, LSU)

Clearly, it was possible for people to see a person in seclusion, and the women could not be sure that their privacy was being respected. There may have been visitors from outside the hospital at the front desk who could witness the woman in various states of undress. On the MSU, there was more privacy for those in seclusion, but it was still possible to witness people being moved into seclusion from the central office window. Here, a client on the MSU described the seclusion room experience:

Rebecca: You were in that blue room?
Sarah: Yes, it's cold as well in there.
Rebecca: What does it feel like being inside there?
Sarah: It's horrible.
Rebecca: Is somebody watching you?
Sarah: Yes staff are watching, in a little room with the window, watching you, observing.
Rebecca: What do they do?
Sarah: They just sit there writing in the yellow book.
Rebecca: And what do you do?
Sarah: Nothing, just banging around.
Rebecca: Do they take off your clothes?
Sarah: No, I just went to sleep after that.

(Interview, client, MSU)

Sarah's experience of being secluded shows that no engagement with staff occurs. Some staff told me that they were discouraged from engaging with clients in seclusion, despite this being a private opportunity where women often find the need to talk and explain the reasons for their behaviour. I argue that this is yet another area where staff/client relationships are maligned and discouraged, and this is rationalised yet again by the suggestion that making it into a positive experience would encourage women's reliance on this coercive method.

Alternatives to seclusion

Many of the clients in my research had ideas about alternative measures which could have been used before seclusion was deployed. Most of the suggestions involved having the opportunity to go to another room away from others to calm down and talk to staff about how they feel:

Rebecca: OK so can you think of anything that might be better for people other than putting them in the seclusion room?

Bonnie: If there's another room away from seclusion, you know like a calm down room, I reckon that they should talk to us and say 'How do you feel, what can we do to help you?' and that.

(Interview, client, LSU)

Staff/client engagement was key when people were suggesting changes to the system. If it is possible for staff to spend time with people before they get to crisis point, then this may reduce the need for coercive measures. Staff members also made similar suggestions, for example:

Dawn: And I think seclusion is good for certain people however, I think we could do with a HDU [high dependency unit] area as well as seclusion because we have in the past used seclusion to try and take people away from the stimulus because they've been up here [gestures height with hand], but perhaps they've not needed to be secluded at that point. They might have done eventually but if they'd carried on in there. So we could do with a high dependency area where perhaps they don't need secluding yet.

(Interview, qualified staff, LSU)

This is pointing to a problem with the use of space on the LSU; if there was another area where people could be moved to away from other clients, then seclusion may not be needed. If it is the need for removal of stimuli that causes seclusion, there should be a better way to do this. Here, a senior member of staff talked about finding alternatives when it was decided that a woman was becoming 'dependent' on seclusion:

Rebecca: I remember you saying that instead of using seclusion as a controlling thing, you did more positive stuff. What did you do?

Karen: Well if someone had been, I think in particular for one client who's moved on now, she was dependent on seclusion seven days a week. I think what we ended up doing was realising that we would take each day as it came, so if she wasn't in seclusion we would do something very positive with her and rewarding with her. So eventually she got it that when she wasn't in seclusion something nice was happening.

Rebecca: Just to get her out of that dependence?

Karen: Just to get her out yes.

Rebecca: And now she's moved on?

Karen: Yes, there are other ways you can do it, there are other ways of keeping them in a sitting restraint and keeping them safe in the HDU, and challenging that, but it depends on the level of aggression. You know sometimes you can get to a stage where you can sit with them for the majority of the day. And that's fine, keeping them out of seclusion.

Rebecca: But that's boring isn't it for everybody?

Karen: Well yes it is but it just stops them getting that dependence of seclusion a lot of the time. Because there's a lot that go into seclusion and then their aggression's gone [claps hands]. Well it doesn't serve a purpose then though does it. Because they're just fighting to get into seclusion and then the fight's gone. So it's about keep working through that fighting and keep – 'You're safe, you're here, we're with you, let's sit in the HDU' and it's about that. And it's a long long long process, sometimes. But sometimes it works, sometimes it doesn't.

(Interview, qualified staff)

Dependence on seclusion was discussed often, as I have shown with the other coercive methods – the alternative being prolonged physical restraint without progression to secluding the person. A few staff talked to me about how people can become dependent on seclusion as it is 'the end of the road' or the final method of containment. It is unclear why this may be, as none of the women spoke about this dependency and none of them told me that they wanted to be or liked being secluded. Nevertheless, it is reasonable to deduce that solitude may occasionally be preferable to communal areas at times of distress, for some people. I argue that gentle positive engagement could be considered to effectively remove the need for seclusion.

Termination of seclusion

There is no denying that a period of seclusion compels the person to appear calm, although what constitutes 'calm' in this environment could be simply a manifestation of defeat and immobility. Some of the women did acknowledge that it helped them to calm down, but it is impossible to deduce whether it was seclusion that prompted this or just removal from the distressing situation.

Karen: I suppose because you just get to know them, you know the signs and you know the triggers and you can see in general presentation, physical presentation. They're not anxious any more, they're not red in the face, they're not shouting and screaming, they're very calm, they're talking to you, they've had some medication. There are occasions when we think they're calm and they come out and we have to put them back in again, but not very often. You just get to know the signs really.

(Interview, qualified staff)

Techniques of power: control of information

Another, more subtle method of controlling people which my research flagged up concerned the directional flow of information. Clients on the unit had reports written about them which followed them from service to service, and this knowledge contributed to how they were treated on admission and, in some ways, throughout their time on the unit, as Stewart illustrated:

Stewart: Unfortunately some of our clients will have had a lifetime in services. We've a young lady who's only just turned 19 and has been in services since she was probably about 12, so all her teenage years into early adulthood has been explicitly documented, she can't blow her nose without it being written down somewhere. So for some people we'll know everything, certainly if they've been in other medium secure units, or services similar to us, they'll very often use the same documents.

(Interview, qualified staff)

The flow of information was one way, however. There were lots of instances of people telling me that they were not given information about things that happened to them, such as the fact that they were moving units or wards, or even as I have already mentioned, the reasons why they were sent to Unit C:

Rebecca: So they didn't tell you that you were coming to live here?
Lorna: I thought I was just coming for a visit. Because if they had told me, I would probably have kicked off in the van. So they said to me, 'You're on a visit' so I wouldn't kick off.

(Interview, client, MSU)

Lorna pointed out that the reason she was not told by her previous service that she was moving to Unit C was because she would have been upset prior to the move, and she admits that she would have acted aggressively if they had told her. This paternalistic filtering of information is a feature in services for learning disabled people, where staff make choices about what to tell people. Ellie also described being moved abruptly and without warning:

Rebecca: When you came here, did people tell you that you were coming here?
Ellie: Not at [Unit], they just, my bags were all ready and that was it, I just came here.
Rebecca: And they didn't tell you where you were going?
Ellie: uh huh, because I had to go to an appointment first and then started in this way.
Rebecca: So how did you feel when you knew you were going somewhere where they hadn't told you?
Ellie: I felt upset, because I didn't say goodbye to my friend.

(Interview, client, LSU)

Notwithstanding the reasons why Ellie was not prepared for the move, the fact that she was lacking in information left her with lasting feelings of regret. Marion was aware that there was a harm-minimisation policy in place for some clients, yet here she pointed out that she was not being allowed to self-harm like other people and not told the reasons why:

Marion: [I know that] other patients' guidelines say they can self-harm and if they can self-harm I don't think that's very fair, I should be able to self-harm as well.

Rebecca: Does it not depend on how you do it?

Marion: I don't know, I've no idea, I couldn't tell you.

Rebecca: So they've not talked to you about it, why you have to be restrained?

Marion: I'm not supposed to hurt myself, but other people do, they say it's in my guidelines. I feel as though I'm flogging a dead horse, I feel it goes in one ear and out the other and over their heads. They're just not listening to me, I can talk to them til I'm black and blue in the face and still they won't listen to me.

Rebecca: Do you get to see your guidelines?

Marion: No.

Rebecca: Who gets to see them then?

Marion: Basically the doctor and the staff.

Rebecca: So staff tell you what's in your guidelines.

Marion: They say that it says in my guidelines that I shouldn't self-harm and they're here to protect me and they're here to look after me.

(Interview, client, LSU)

Marion had been told that she was not allowed to self-harm, yet she saw the harm-minimisation policy being implemented with other clients. Marion has not been informed about why the policy cannot be used with her, and what she would have to do to have this made available to her. Of course, decisions could have been made about Marion's current state of mind to which I had not been party, but the reasons for these decisions should have been made clear to Marion.

It seems that the control of information in such a paternalistic way is particular to learning disability services (e.g. Tuffrey-Wijne et al., 2009), and there do seem to be clear reasons for not giving the women in this study certain items of information, for example to mitigate feelings of distress about inevitable events. However, this detail again reveals the contradiction between the discourse of policy (control, choice, information) and the reality of practice.

Resistance

Foucault (1980) famously observed that there cannot be power without resistance, and although resistance from the women in my study was still determined by the system to be within narrow parameters, it undeniably existed. Whether the resistances were effective is debatable. There are instances of resistance to special observation in the literature, most notably in Harker-Longton and Fish's (2002) study where the research participant pointed out that even having six staff watching her would not be enough to stop her from self-harming. If passivity is the final goal of the institution, then these coercive methods are not usually working. This may be why the staff continue to rationalise clients' behaviour as provocative, with intent to bring about these measures, because clients continue to behave in ways which lead to them. If clients are not exposed to instances where they can communicate their wishes and challenge the system, then they will never find out how to have an influence on their futures. As Sullivan and Mullen (2012:295) claim, the staff/client relationship 'is not a relationship of equality, nor of choice, nor consent. The only real power available to the patient/prisoner is the power to disrupt and refuse.' Encouragingly, this was not always the case at Unit C. Here is an example of one woman managing to resist the status quo in a successful way (I have called her Jane in this instance as the excerpt contains information which could identify her):

Jane: I had good news, I never told you no. I went to um, ward round on Wednesday. I told [psychiatrist], I said, 'Hold on, stop there,' and I stopped him. And I said, 'You know that crime I done,' he said, 'Yes.' I said, 'I not done it in, hold on, I done it in [town 1] not in [town 2].' I asked him again, I said 'Am I allowed to go to [town 2] to visit [my husband]?' and he turned round and said, 'Yes, with two staff.'

Rebecca: That's brilliant!

Jane: And I was so happy!

Rebecca: I can imagine.

Jane: I was! And I've no idea, I don't know why I said that.

Rebecca: So you've never asked before?

Jane: No, and now, I asked. I did, I stuck up for myself.

(Interview, client, LSU)

Here, Jane points out how she managed to influence her circumstances in a positive way, by 'sticking up for herself' rather than by using what is considered to be bad behaviour.

There were many instances of clients describing their resistance to the rules by using self-harming or destructive behaviour, for example:

Annie: I had an incident when I were punching walls and head-butting the bar in the garden I were throwing chairs, trying to smash the windows with chairs because I were so angry.

(Interview, client, LSU)

Clearly, the institution is not making 'docile bodies' – that not only do what the staff want but in precisely the way they want it done (Foucault, 1979:138).

However, there are narrow parameters for resistance and rules that seem intrusive can provoke intense reactions, as Brenda describes here:

Brenda: I do get angry, I still lash out and I tend to when I'm getting restrained, I tend to kick me feet. And not purposely, I have made the occasional contact.

Rebecca: Why do you think you get so angry?

Brenda: I don't know, it's just little things. Like to other people it might mean nothing getting the door closed but to me it means a lot, it's peace, it's privacy. Sometimes when [client] goes to her bedroom, you've got staff sitting outside watching her and it's a nightmare she decides all of a sudden, she'll say "I'm bored, can I play music?' And it's like a disco in her room and I just want to close my door.

(Interview, client, MSU)

Brenda's door was a symbol of privacy for her. She liked to go to her room and write about her day, but noise from other rooms disturbed her. Due to her previous self-harm, she wasn't allowed to keep her door closed when she was in her room, but this was a rule with which she did not agree. However, this kind of resistance always worked against clients and resulted in further coercive measures being used, or incentives being lost. Another method of resistance which was described by some staff was making false allegations against staff:

Iona: One of the things she did tell me that was hilarious, she used to actually make a lot of allegations that the staff were coming into her room at night with various vegetables and performing sexual acts on her and they'd have to obviously take it seriously and take it forward and that and, that was quite common. When she moved into community she actually very seriously said, 'You know I used to make all those allegations, I can't do that anymore.' I said, 'Why not?' She said, 'Well they have to call the police and if you're not telling the truth they don't take it very kindly.'

(Interview, qualified staff)

Clients' efforts to gain some sort of power or control, were often conceived in terms of 'manipulation'; for example self-harm can be seen by staff as a power issue, in the form of attention seeking, or as clients' attempts to have some sort of control over their bodies when they are lacking in control in other areas (Fish, 2000). Some women's ongoing attempts to influence staff were often talked about as 'manipulative':

Iona: [She was manipulative in that she] would play me off against everybody else, the female staff, not the male staff, just the female staff. It's 'Iona gives me this, she gives me that, Iona does this for me, does that for me.' Then she would encourage the whispering and the [laugh] bitchiness that goes with women, you know. The inability really to express themselves to each other, and having to sort of analyse it from a nasty point of view really I suppose. Until I confronted them and said, 'Every time I come in you stop talking, what's going on?' And then it all came out, and it was very believable. Nothing [client] had said about me was actually true, but . . . I'd say to her 'Yes, that's a fantastic idea.' You know what I mean? But I didn't do anything different for her than I would for any of the other women that I worked with.

(Interview, qualified staff)

Iona talked about the woman causing trouble between staff as a way to get what she wanted, and how she herself was treated by other staff because they thought she was offering preferential treatment to a client. As we have seen with women diagnosed with BPD, there was a very real sense of clients causing trouble between staff, and staff policing other staff's relationships with clients. This was a thread among some of the clients' discussions also, for example when Annie was talking about another client using self-harm to gain attention:

Annie: Because [Jane] does it, every time [Tanya] does something and ends up on a level or when the certain shift is on tonight, [Jane] wants to be on a level so she can be with one person, then two people and no one else can have any of the attention, she's got to have the attention.

(Interview, client, LSU)

Annie suggested that Jane used self-harm to take staff's attention away from Tanya, who also self-harmed. So, it is evident that any attempts to gain control or influence staff on behalf of clients become construed as 'manipulation', and this idea has become internalised by clients. Len Bowers points out that a 'completely normal and natural emotional response to being detained against your will is to be angry, and consider those who operate the detention system as your enemies' (Bowers, 2003:330). In agreement with this, Iona suggested that the organisation may play a role in manipulative behaviour by taking away all power:

Iona: [Clients can be manipulative because] I don't think we take empowering roles with a lot of people, we tend to take that power away and that control in their lives as they do in most places like this.

It seems that craving for attention is exacerbated by the restrictive system, although some staff managed to accept and work with this behaviour. Iona went on to say that in some sense, letting people take the lead can be productive in the staff/client relationship, but she also acknowledged how difficult this is:

Iona: It was a quirky relationship really from somebody who really made me laugh and made me think about life a bit differently, and not to get upset about it, not to get upset about working with people who want to manipulate you, be manipulated to some extent . . . I know I've used that word quite a lot and I don't think it's truly what I mean to say, manipulated. I've not really thought about it in an analytical point of view but that's how it feels when you're on the receiving end of it.

(Interview, qualified staff)

Iona pointed out that from the staff's point of view, feeling manipulated can be unpleasant and upsetting; however, for clients, there seemed to be few ways to challenge the rules without using 'manipulation'. Jackie's forward-thinking idea was to have a collaborative forum for negotiation, so that people are not just 'done to':

Jackie: And ideally they would be – maybe not initially collaborative, because there's something about when somebody comes in the door you have to have some guidelines as to how to respond to somebody, but then as you go along, I think there's something about when women particularly are calmer or they're in a good space, there's something about it being a collaborative process and giving them some responsibility. So you know like this the other week 'how best can we help you at these times?' So it's not just the staff 'doing to', it's something about, and I suppose that's where the self-harm stuff has come, the guidelines being more collaborative, rather than 'doing to', so: 'These are your guidelines that we've devised and we're going to [be] applying to you when you're like this.'

(Interview, qualified staff)

Jackie's ideas about collaborative planning and asking women how they would prefer to be treated in times of anger and distress, are more about sharing the power and control, bringing to mind the disability activists' mantra 'nothing about us without us'. I argue that attention from staff is a legitimate requirement in such units, and if this was freely given, behaviour which is interpreted as 'attention seeking' and 'manipulative' would be considered an indication that extra support is needed and the power struggles which have been described would be re-evaluated. As I have shown, at Unit C, the available means of resistance were few, and were often comprehended as 'manipulative' which resulted in further constraints being placed on the women.

Yates's points out that employees of service agencies are encouraged to think constantly about values but 'rarely about power relations between service users and support workers – *except* where service users are deemed to behave in a "manipulative" fashion, in which case *they* are seen to attempt power play over *us*' (Yates, 2005:234, emphasis in original). Bowers proposes that this is part of the 'therapy vs control' dilemma which is experienced by staff (Bowers, 2003:331). Bowers suggests that manipulation should be considered normal behaviour that is a result of a serious imbalance of power, as resistance to this power (See also Powell, 2001).

Often on Unit C, resistance in the form of aggression was attributed to gender, impairment or past experiences of women, and context was overlooked. It could be argued that if context was seen as central, more emphasis would be placed on post-incident debriefing. Although Unit C used 'community meetings' for this purpose, often the discussion would take place a few days after the incident.

Conclusion

In this chapter, I have argued that coercive methods for behaviour management should be investigated using concepts of power and control. Clients in Unit C pointed out the unpleasantness of coercive methods from both staff and client perspectives, and they emphasised the damage it could do to the therapeutic relationship. There were many opportunities being missed for discussion and resolution of conflict.

Although Foucault's theorisation of the Panopticon (Foucault, 1979) as a method to instil discipline and self-regulation described surveillance as faceless and unverifiable, surveillance at Unit C was embodied, as in McCorkel's (2003) ethnographic study, where observer and observed knew each other. McCorkel (2003:65) theorised that this embodiment 'solidified' the power of staff, and this power enabled them to undermine clients' peer relationships and use rule breaking as indications of deviancy. It seems that the continual and ongoing deployment of these practices means that although a 'total institution' in Goffman's terms, Unit C is not actuating 'docile bodies' as suggested by Foucault to be the institutional aim. This is despite the use of all of the measures designed to cause clients to self-direct, and could be considered to be an expression of the strength that has got these women through the bad times they have described.

Although much of the resistance on Unit C was not productive or helpful for the women, I saw some occasions where it was. My argument is that resistance, if seen in context as meaningful and significant, can be constructive. Although it is important not to single out people with learning disabilities as dissimilar from others who are detained in residential services, it is equally important to observe the particularities of services designated as for this group, who have services and policies designed for them on the strength of their impairments. This chapter demonstrates how learning disabled people are perceived and treated as in need of controlling, in terms of their movements, information they are given, and choices they can make. This controlling treatment often begins in early life and people adapt ways of being which fulfil their needs in the short term, such as the resistances to control that we have seen here. Perhaps if learning disabled people were respected as equal in society, this would be reflected in services and the therapeutic relationship would be based more on shared values and mutual respect.

Notes

1 A portion of this chapter has been published as: Fish, R., and Hatton, C. (2017). Gendered experiences of physical restraint on locked wards for women. *Disability and Society*, 32(6), 708–809. DOI: http://dx.doi.org/10.1080/09687599.2017.1329711
2 Bank staff are provided by an agency and are used on an ad-hoc basis to cover periods of short-staffing. They may not have any prior experience of working with the clients.

Bibliography

Aitken, G. & Noble, K. (2001). Violence and violation: women and secure settings. *Feminist Review*, 68(1), 68–88.

Aiyegbusi, A. (2002). Nursing interventions and future directions with women in secure services. *Forensic Focus*, 19, 136–150.Barron, K. (2002). Who am I? Women with learning difficulties (re) constructing their self-identity. *Scandinavian Journal of Disability Research*, 4, 58–79.

Becker, D. (1997). *Through the looking glass: Women and borderline personality disorder*. Boulder, CO: Westview Press.

Bowers, L. (2003). Manipulation: searching for an understanding. *Journal of Psychiatric and Mental Health Nursing*, 10(3), 329–334.

Bowlby, J. (1977). The making and breaking of affectional bonds: I: Aetiology and psychopathology in the light of attachment theory: An expanded version of the Fiftieth Maudsley Lecture, delivered before the Royal College of Psychiatrists, 19 November 1976. *The British Journal of Psychiatry*, 130, 201–210.

Bowlby, J. (2005). *A secure base: Clinical applications of attachment theory*. New York: Routledge.

Bowles, N., Dodds, P., Hackney, D., Sunderland, C., & Thomas, P. (2002). Formal observations and engagement: A discussion paper. *Journal of Psychiatric and Mental Health Nursing*, 9, 255–260.

Breeze, J. A., & Repper, J. (1998). Struggling for control: The care experiences of "difficult" patients in mental health services. *Journal of Advanced Nursing*, 28, 1301–1311.

Brown, J. S., & Tooke, S. K. (1992). On the seclusion of psychiatric patients. *Social Science & Medicine*, 35, 711–721.

Chamberlin, J. (1985). An ex-patient's response to Soliday. *Journal of Nervous and Mental Disease*, 173, 288–289.

Chan, J. (2012). Is it time to drop the term "challenging behaviour"? *Learning Disability Practice*, 15, 36–38.

Clements, J., Clare, I., & Ezelle, L. (1995). Real men, real women, real lives? Gender issues in learning disabilities and challenging behaviour. *Disability & Society*, 10, 425–436.

Crick, N. R., & Grotpeter, J. K. (1995). Relational aggression, gender, and social-psychological adjustment. *Child Development*, 66, 710–722.

Cullerton-Sen, C., Cassidy, A. R., Murray-Close, D., Cicchetti, D., Crick, N. R., & Rogosch, F. A. (2008). Childhood maltreatment and the development of relational and physical aggression: The importance of a gender-informed approach. *Child Development*, 79, 1736–1751.

Cutcliffe, J., & Barker, P. (2002). Considering the care of the suicidal client and the case for "engagement and inspiring hope" or "observations". *Journal of Psychiatric and Mental Health Nursing*, 9, 611–621.

Department of Health. (2007). *Mental Health Act: Code of practice*. London: HMSO.

Duperouzel, H. (2008). "It's OK for people to feel angry": The exemplary management of imminent aggression. *Journal of Intellectual Disabilities*, 12, 295–307.

Duperouzel, H., & Fish, R. (2008). Why couldn't I stop her? Self injury: The views of staff and clients in a medium secure unit. *British Journal of Learning Disabilities*, 36, 59–65.

Duperouzel, H., & Fish, R. (2010). Hurting no-one else's body but your own: People with intellectual disability who self injure in a forensic service. *Journal of Applied Research in Intellectual Disabilities*, 23, 606–615.

Emerson, E. (2001). *Challenging behaviour: Analysis and intervention in people with severe intellectual disabilities*. Cambridge: Cambridge University Press.

Fish, R. (2000). Working with people who harm themselves in a forensic learning disability service: Experiences of direct care staff. *Journal of Learning Disabilities*, 4, 193.

Fish, R. & Culshaw, E. (2005). "The last resort? Staff and client perspectives on physical intervention." *Journal of Intellectual Disabilities*, 9(2): 93–107.

Fish, R., & Duperouzel, H. (2008). Just another day dealing with wounds: Self-injury and staff-client relationships. *Learning Disability Practice*, 11, 12–15.

Foucault, M. (1979). *Discipline and punish: The birth of the prison*. New York: Pantheon

Foucault, M. (1980). *Power/knowledge: Selected interviews and other writings, 1972–1977*. New York: Random House.

Gilburt, H., Rose, D., & Slade, M. (2008). The importance of relationships in mental health care: A qualitative study of service users' experiences of psychiatric hospital admission in the UK. *BMC Health Services Research*, 8, 92.

Harker-Longton, W., & Fish, R. (2002)."Cutting doesn't make you die": One woman's views on the treatment of her self-injurious behaviour. *Journal of Intellectual Disabilities*, 6, 137–151.

Herman, J. (1997). *Trauma and recovery: The aftermath of violence – from domestic abuse to political terror*. New York: Basic Books.

Hoekstra, T., Lendemeijer, H., & Jansen, M. (2004). Seclusion: The inside story. *Journal of Psychiatric and Mental Health Nursing*, 11, 276–283.

James, M., & Warner, S. (2005). Coping with their lives – women, learning disabilities, self-harm and the secure unit: A Q-methodological study. *British Journal of Learning Disabilities*, 33, 120–127.

Kendall, K. (2004). Female offenders or alleged offenders with developmental disabilities: A critical overview. In *Offenders with developmental disabilities*. W. R. Lindsay, J. L. Taylor and P. Sturmey. Oxford, Wiley: 265–288.

Kleinberg, I., & Scior, K. (2014). The impact of staff and service user gender on staff responses towards adults with intellectual disabilities who display aggressive behaviour. *Journal of Intellectual Disability Research*, 58, 110–124.

Liebling, H., Chipchase, H., & Velangi, R. (1997). Why do women harm themselves? – Surviving special hospitals. *Feminism & Psychology*, 7, 427–435.

Mason, J., & Scior, K. (2004). "Diagnostic overshadowing" amongst clinicians working with people with intellectual disabilities in the UK. *Journal of Applied Research in Intellectual Disabilities*, 17, 85–90.

Mccorkel, J. A. (2003). Embodied surveillance and the gendering of punishment. *Journal of Contemporary Ethnography*, 32, 41–76.

Mcsherry, B. (2017). Regulating seclusion and restraint in health care settings: The promise of the convention on the rights of persons with disabilities. *International Journal of Law and Psychiatry*, 53, 39–44.

National Institute for Health and Care Excellence. (2011). *Self harm: Longer-term management*. NICE guidance (CG133). London: National Institute for Health and Care Excellence.

Oddie, S., & Ousley, L. (2007). Assessing burn-out and occupational stressors in a medium secure service. *The British Journal of Forensic Practice*, 9, 32–48.

Parry-Crooke, G., & Stafford, P. (2009). *My life: In safe hands?* London: Metropolitan University.

Phillips, D. (2005). Embodied narratives: Control, regulation and bodily resistance in the life course of women with learning difficulties. In D. Goodley & G. Van Hove (Eds.), *Another disability studies reader? People with learning disabilities & a disabling world*, (pp. 133–150). Antwerp: Garant.

Powell, J. (2001). Women in British special hospitals: A sociological approach. *Sincronia: Journal of Social Sciences and Humanities*, 5, 1–14.

Secker, J., Benson, A., Balfe, E., Lipsedge, M., Robinson, S., & Walker, J. (2004). Understanding the social context of violent and aggressive incidents on an inpatient unit. *Journal of Psychiatric and Mental Health Nursing*, 11, 172–178.

Sequeira, H., & Halstead, S. (2001). Is it meant to hurt, is it? *Violence Against Women*, 7, 462–476.

Smith, H. P., & Power, J. (2014). Themes underlying self-injurious behavior in prison: Gender convergence and divergence. *Journal of Offender Rehabilitation*, 53, 273–299.

Sullivan, D. H. & Mullen, P.E. (2012). Mental Health and Human Rights in Secure Settings. Mental Health and Human Rights: Vision, Praxis, and Courage. In M. Dudley, D. Silove and F. Gale. Oxford, Oxford University Press: 283–296

Tuffrey-Wijne, I., Bernal, J., Hubert, J., Butler, G., & Hollins, S. (2009). People with learning disabilities who have cancer: An ethnographic study. *British Journal of General Practice*, 59, 503–509.

Veltkamp, E., Nijman, H., Stolker, J., Frigge, K., Dries, P., & Bowers, L. (2008). Patients' preferences for seclusion or forced medication in acute psychiatric emergency in the Netherlands. *Psychiatric Services*, 59, 209–211.

Wilcox, E., Finlay, W., & Edmonds, J. (2006). His brain is totally different: An analysis of care-staff explanations of aggressive challenging behaviour and the impact of gendered discourses. *British Journal of Social Psychology*, 45, 197–216.

Williams, J., Scott, S., & Waterhouse, S. (2001). Mental health services for "difficult" women: Reflections on some recent developments. *Feminist Review*, 68, 89–104.

Yates, S. (2005). Truth, power, and ethics in care services for people with learning difficulties. In S. Tremain (Ed.), *Foucault and the government of disability* (pp. 65–77). Michigan: University of Michigan Press.

6 Moving on

Progression through services

Undoubtedly, evidence of progression through services is important to both staff and clients. Literature relating to progression and rehabilitation in the field of learning disabilities centres mainly on particular empirical tools used to evaluate treatment programmes and analyse risk, and recidivism rates in the longer term (Barron et al., 2002). There is very little research describing people's views of potential outcomes from using forensic services. This is where the literature diverges from that of mental health rehabilitation, where the intention is to stimulate 'recovery'. Originating in the survivor movement, the concept of recovery has been adopted by service user activists as a way to describe the reclamation of a meaningful life, even though the person might still be experiencing symptoms (McWade, 2014). There is some debate over whether recovery is a meaningful aspiration, indeed whether it should be relegated to the medical or individual model of disability (Beresford, 2005). Because recovery can be defined in different ways, and refers to both process and outcome, there is some confusion about which dimensions of recovery should matter, as I will discuss.

Recently, theories of recovery in psychiatric services have moved away from the absence of 'mental illness' symptoms to more subjective and holistic parameters (Schrank and Slade, 2007). Resnick et al. (2005) used personal experiences in general psychiatric services to construct an empirical conceptualisation of recovery, and from this proposed four dimensions of recovery: the capacity to feel empowered in one's life; self-perception and knowledge of one's condition; satisfaction with one's quality of life, and hope and optimism for the future. Mancini (2008) grouped together themes conducive to recovery from a meta-analysis of mental health literature and added the following conditions to this list: autonomy and self-agency, supportive relationships and enhanced role functioning. Mancini's paper is calling for a 'self-determination' model of recovery, which relies on three human needs (autonomy, competence and relatedness to others). Although these models are extremely relevant to the women in my study, it is easy to see that these dimensions are not easy to nurture in forensic services, mainly due to the perceived lack of control and choice (Simpson and Penney, 2011; Turton et al., 2011). Compulsory care restricts liberty and autonomous decision-making, particularly in a setting for learning disabled people. As described earlier in this book, forensic clients are more likely to have had traumatic past experiences which can lead to diminished community and family supports. Additionally, as outlined in Chapter 4, supportive relationships between clients are often not encouraged.

Although recovery in forensic services is more difficult to establish, Ward and Brown (2004) describe a model of recovery they refer to as the 'Good Lives Model' of offender rehabilitation, which replaces a focus on criminality and risk with one which looks towards a future of well-being and motivation. The person is included in discussions about their future, and the tasks they can fulfil to work towards recovery. Given the diverse nature of women's pathways into Unit C, this type of approach should, in my view, appeal to this service. However, it seemed that 'progression' was discussed rather than recovery, and the criteria for progression, although planned using information about the individual, focussed on reduction of current problematic behaviour. Travers observed a similar phenomenon in psychiatric services and claimed that this is due to women's admission to forensic services as 'determined by enduring behavioural disturbances in other residential environments' (2013:69). These behavioural disturbances are seen to require an environment with greater restrictions in order to modify them, therefore behavioural stability determines progression for women in these services (see also Aiyegbusi, 2002; Alexander et al., 2011). What is important, however, is how do staff and clients perceive concepts of progression, and how does progression happen?

Concepts of progression

Progression held different meanings for staff and clients on Unit C, depending on the reason for admission. I did not have access to any official documents or discussions concerning progression; my interest was in how people understood and experienced the phenomenon in relation to each client. The overall deliberation about progression was about enacting or producing some form of change, as evidenced here:

Adele: It's not that you can change the person, you change the behaviour and the way they behave in a particular given situation, but first of all they have to recognise that that's how they behave in the given situation. And that's the hard bit, is getting people to actually say, 'Oh yeah, that's what I do and I don't want to do it any more and therefore I'll try and do this instead.' Once they've got to that point and they can really try, they may be able to then start learning better ways of coping so that they don't hurt themselves or others, or replicate difficult relationships that they've previously had [any more]. So no, you can't inherently change the personality, but you can learn different ways of coping with it.

(Interview, qualified staff)

Although I found it encouraging that staff did consider the women's past experiences as contributing to their current circumstances, I also felt that this discourse left very little space to talk about positives, such as good family and peer relationships, and skills and resources that women already had and could build on. There was evidence, however, that pasts were being used to contextualise behaviour and to work with the women to find out reasons, such as in Stewart's account:

Stewart: No matter what we do we're never going to cure people. The stuff that's – certainly in [client's] case – the stuff that's gone on, we're never going to get rid of and she'll never be okay with that, it'll always cause her problems. She's damaged now, unfortunately. As lovely as she is, her life is damaged by what's happened and again, all we can do is make her feel safe, give her better coping strategies, but at times – those aren't going to work all the time, so we've not to be too hard on ourselves when things go wrong. We'll go back to the drawing board, re-design things again, get her involved: 'Why was it that you hit that person? Was it something they said?'

(Interview, qualified staff)

Stewart refers to redesigning care in response to the client, something which aligns his practice with the social model of disability, insofar as he is modifying his care in respect to her. This shows that when staff become aware of women's pasts, they are considered to be static and women are considered to be damaged as a result. Importantly however, Stewart shows that keeping this knowledge in mind can sometimes be productive. Debate on this topic is divided, some authors consider looking to people's pasts to be problematic; for example some research has found that services' knowledge of a client's past abuse adversely informs conceptions of risk (Pollack, 2007; Adshead, 2011). Conversely, some authors advocate looking to the past in terms of treatment, but in practice, found that past trauma is not taken into account due to services applying a medical model in treatment (Brackenridge and Morrissey, 2010; Rossiter, 2012). My argument is that pasts should be taken into account, but alongside and together with individuals' futures.

When clients were telling me their ideas about how they could 'move on' in the service, I noted a number of themes: taking back responsibility, proving success in arranged relationships and acceptance of the regime on the unit. These were interrelated and complex, but all were models of progression which had been determined by staff.

Taking back responsibility: 'Keep off my levels'

Taking responsibility and gaining trust were prominent in discussions about progression on Unit C. For example, Dawn told me about Jane who, after years of special observation, was considered to be progressing extremely well and would soon be moving into the community:

Dawn: Um when she came here she had, I think it was, two very serious incidents where she um tried to strangle herself and was cyanosed, and lips had turned blue and she had to go to hospital. And then she was such a high suicide risk because it was all that she wanted to do. So she was placed on a level and then every time we tried to take her off a level, years ago, every single time we tried, she'd make an attempt at suicide. So it was because she'd made an attempt at suicide, after that people became so scared to take her off this level that it became a way of life. But then she became so dependent on the level it was like, it wasn't serving a purpose [pause]. I think as she became more well, it wasn't serving the purpose to stop her trying to kill herself because she'd calmed, not got over it but kind of she was a bit better than she had been and that wasn't the main thing [in her life]. But then she felt like she needed that security blanket of that person, when you're used to having someone with you 24 hours a day, for them suddenly to take it away it's just a shock to the system isn't it?

Rebecca: So how did you do it?

Dawn: [Hums and laughs exasperatedly] Very hard! We started off allowing her to go in the toilet on her own and we'd stand outside the door and just have voice contact with her.

Rebecca: Before that you were watching her on the loo and everything?

Dawn: Yes, shower, toilet, bed literally 24 hours a day she didn't do anything without a staff member watching her do it or a staff member with her.

Rebecca: So it was just gradually doing it then.

Dawn: Very gradual, very slowly, very gradual and Jane can ask any time, she has two face-to-face contacts a day so she speaks to someone in the morning, and at night-time about how she's feeling, whether she's settled, does she think she's well enough to be off a level or not. And if at any point she's feeling a bit unsettled or doesn't feel particularly well she can just say 'I don't feel right today, can I be on my level?' and staff will say 'Yes, fine' and they'll just re-implement it. But then a couple of hours later if she's picked up say 'Jane do you feel alright now?' and reduce it straight away again. So she's in control and it's really helped.

(Interview, qualified staff)

Dawn spoke about how clients become 'dependent' on interventions such as special observation, an idea which I discussed in the previous chapter. Jane is described as needing staff as safety, as a 'security blanket' and that having control of her situation has helped her to come through this. Rather than conceptualising this as compelling the client to obey the rules, Dawn describes the process as one of handing over control, when this control had been originally in staff's hands. This process of handing over control must have felt very risky at the time for staff. Jane herself told me about this situation:

Rebecca: So when we're talking about moving on, what kinds of things do you think you can do to move on?

Jane: Well keep off my levels, just keep to yourself and work hard and talk to the staff when you're down. Yes.

Rebecca:	So will you tell me about these levels? Because you've done really well getting off your levels.
Jane:	Well at first I got like five minutes in my room, then ten minutes, and in ward round I says 'Can I have half an hour, just staff stay with me while I'm asleep.' I've gone off that, and then I've gone off at daytime and I'm just off it now.
Rebecca:	So you don't ever get put back on it?
Jane:	Oh yes if I feel that I'm down I'll say 'Can I go onto a level 3?' Is it level 3? Sommat like that.
Rebecca:	Yes, and when you were on a level . . .
Jane:	Ooh it were awful, no privacy or anything.

(Interview, client, LSU)

Although Jane stressed that she did not like being on a level, most of the women told me that they like having the company of staff when they are not too busy. Perhaps Jane's perceived dependence on the levels was because she enjoyed the companionship, even though the accompanying surveillance felt punitive.

This situation demonstrates the inconsistencies on Unit C my research revealed. Women stated their dislike of the coercive methods, yet staff explain women's actions as trying to bring these about. Jane's story shows, however, that it is possible for women to keep themselves safe.

Success in arranged relationships: 'Prove that you can live with someone'

Elaine's concept of progression was being able to live successfully with another person. Elaine had to live by herself for a number of years previous to this. She told me that the reason she was in the unit was to 'get better and move on':

Rebecca:	How do you think you're moving on? What's helping?
Elaine:	Well I am moving on now because I'm living with someone now, living with [name] and I'm getting on alright with [name] all the time.
Rebecca:	You're getting on with her? Is it hard work trying to get on?
Elaine:	No I'm getting used to it now, to live with someone, yes I'm getting used to it now . . . [You have to just] prove that you can behave and prove that you can live with someone.

(Interview, client, LSU)

Elaine's perception of how she could progress was to have tolerance for living with another client. She had been moved in with a woman who was described to me by staff as 'resilient' and 'laid back' in order to help Elaine learn to live with others. This arrangement must have felt like a big step at the time; as we have seen in Chapter 4, living in close proximity to others who are at different stages in their progression is not easy. The progress that Elaine has made was due to the sustained support from staff for both women throughout the process and had been successful for a number of months when I arrived, demonstrating that concepts of progression are individually planned, tackling one aspect of the client's rehabilitation at a time.

Relationships between clients are not always encouraged when they become too close, and according to Holland and Meddis (1993), this is because of the importance placed on staff/client relationships. Indeed on Unit C, stable staff/client relationships were used as markers of progress, and although staff tried to make sense of the aggression they sometimes encountered, this often proved to be quite difficult. Some staff's concepts of progression tended to focus on absence of aggression and use of anger management techniques. However, staff did accept that progression takes time. Monica, for example focussed on relational factors as indicators of results:

> *Monica:*   I think there's a general lack of acceptance that we're not going to make giant leaps with these women overnight. And I think we should celebrate small wins, whereas I think we want to sometimes 'love them better'. We think if we're never-endingly kind and lovely they're going to be better and it's not the case. It's still nice to be kind and have unconditional positive regard, but I think as staff you've to be very resilient and you can take the knock backs and you can take the 'I've been nice to you for 13 hours and you've just punched me as I've walked out.' I think you need to be able to accept that and think, 'She's probably done it because of whatever'. I think staff get so frustrated and they come in every day and try so hard and don't see massive results. But I think they have too much of an expectation to see massive results.
>
> *(Interview, staff member)*

Monica described how difficult it is to work with somebody every day and not expect 'results'. Being able to imagine a reason for the 'knock backs' or aggression is very important to her. She talked about 'Unconditional Positive Regard' as important,[1] but ultimately the search for reasons and understandings for clients' behaviour as most important for staff 'resilience'. Monica went on to say that perhaps the reasons for lack of progression are more complex:

> *Monica:*   It's only what I think, that women don't seem to move on very quickly. And I think with certain people you expect to see massive wins, and people get frustrated, 'What are we doing for her?' and I'll say, 'Well maybe she's not assaulted anyone for eight weeks, so you've not discharged her, but she's not assaulted anyone for eight weeks.' Previously who was maybe assaulting someone every day. But they don't celebrate that. It's like, 'Well we haven't dropped her supervision levels, or we haven't moved her off this ward' . . . Sometimes you will get a good win where they'll move on, do really well, get resettled and it's a success story. But I think you've just got to keep re-checking the reasons why you came into this work and what you're wanting to achieve

and I think you have to be resilient and I think you have to be quite a robust character or else it can wear you down.

(Interview, qualified staff)

Monica acknowledged that progression is often a slow process, and explained how staff may feel when a woman is not progressing, but she also implicated the organisational regime for this lack of progression. The example she gave is that a woman who was often aggressive did not assault anyone for eight weeks, yet her circumstances did not change quickly enough in response to this, so neither the woman nor the staff figure this as a 'result'. Monica construed progression in terms of behavioural stability here, a common interpretation in Unit C. This is a gendered concept of progression which literature states is more often applied in women's services (Alexander et al., 2011).

Acceptance of regime: 'Do whatever we have to'

Another conception of progression involved notions of 'acceptance' of staff decisions and the institutional regime. John told me about Annie's recent progress. She had been more tolerant about changes of plans and had not been aggressive. John was pleased about this, but he was concerned about the lack of ways to report positive behaviour due to the systems in place focussing on problematic ones:

Rebecca: When you say she's been good one particular day what do you mean?

John: Accepting things. The main one with Annie is she asks for things a lot, very manipulative. Before, if you said no she could get very aggressive about it and lately I find she's been accepting things and not reacting, and waiting for a solution to the problem, where before she would just react and either self-harm or get aggressive.

Rebecca: So you feel like she's moving forward?

John: I personally do, yes I think she is. And Annie herself will tell you, when she was on the MSU [Medium Secure Unit] they had a lot more structure over there and she likes structure, they need to feel, they need boundaries and she'll tell you herself, 'I need boundaries.' Give her too much and then that's when it starts, she gets too much if you know what I mean, it's overload.

Rebecca: I wanted to ask about all the paperwork that you have to fill in and you were saying that you wrote something really good about Annie, but that will just get glossed over.

John: Glossed over yes, I find that when they do the ward round reports they look at the trips out and the bad behaviours, because nobody has got the time to go through the daily notes, every daily notes. I personally think that when they've had an exceptional day it gets overlooked and maybe the people who do the notes who work it out could do a note or a flag up for it. Personally I think that.

(Interview, staff member)

John put forward that Annie's improvement in behaviour was due to boundaries and structure in her life, which he saw as something she did not have before she came to the service. John felt that opportunities to report and reflect on this improvement were lacking. This is similar to what Monica was saying about the lack of 'celebration' of achievements and reflects the focus on negatives within the processes of the service.

Most of the women talked about their future in terms of when they 'get out' – Kate told me her detailed plans for the future and this led into a discussion about how to 'get out', which again involved acceptance of the institutional routine:

Rebecca: Do you know when you're going to "get out"?
Kate: No not yet. We just have to do what the staff tell us to do because at the end of the day they've only got our best interests at heart. Do whatever they say, don't refuse to take our medications, do whatever we have to do, behave, don't go against our treatment and care plans by refusing medication or refusing to eat. Don't refuse work because that can delay you going even if you refuse your work, that can delay you. Don't refuse work, go even if you don't like it until you can get it changed, stuff like that.
Rebecca: So if you do all these things correctly, what's going to happen?
Kate: Well obviously we'll have to do all this for like three months. Non-stop.
Rebecca: And will they tell you that you're doing things good?
Kate: Yes they'll tell us that we're going in the right direction. Like last year they spoke to me about [moving] in July. Beginning of October I were gone, and that's because I were doing everything right. And they will say to us every now and again the doctors, 'You're doing well, carry on and you won't have long left.'

Kate's beliefs about progression included 'doing everything right': complying with treatment, including medication and making sure she goes to work even if she does not want to. This progress had been flagged up to her as positive by the psychiatrists, and she felt that she had seen the results of her progress in the past. Kate went on to tell me that she felt that she was progressing herself, due to the therapy she had received helping her to deal with her past experiences:

Rebecca: When you said you've got rid of all those bad things, how do you feel you've worked through them?
Kate: Yes, it took a hell of a long time but we have we've worked through it together.
Rebecca: And where do you think they've gone, just gone forever?
Kate: They haven't gone forever, they're still there now and again, but . . .
Rebecca: But you can deal with them?
Kate: Yes, like it's in my mind now, I'm thinking about it now while I'm talking to you.
Rebecca: Oh, I'm sorry,

Kate: No, it doesn't upset me anymore, it doesn't upset me . . . It's like I was saying to [name], the new staff. I told her why I'm in here and why I were in care and all that lot and I said, 'If you ever want to ask a question about my background, just ask me.' I said, 'I will answer your question but it won't be just a yes or no, it'll be a full answer.'

(Interview, client, LSU)

Despite Kate's claim that therapy has helped her to deal with her past, it seemed that personal notions of progression and recovery (such as being able to talk about the past) were sometimes at odds with the organisation's. The women did not have a clear idea of how their progress was measured and what they had to achieve in order to move on. Sometimes it seemed that expectations were too high. In this revealing example Tanya told me how difficult it was to interpret:

Rebecca: What's counted as a good day?
Tanya: When you don't do anything wrong. You have to be happy.
Rebecca: What's 'wrong'? Not shouting?
Tanya: Not being quiet either.
Rebecca: You're not allowed to be quiet?
Tanya: You're not allowed to be quiet because they'll think you're 'on one' [sulking].
Rebecca: So how can you convince them you are having a good day then?
Tanya: You have to be talkative and happy.
Rebecca: Right, that's quite a hard [task] . . .

(Interview, client, LSU)

Tanya describes the almost impossible situation of trying to convince staff that she is having a 'good day'. A woman is judged as moving on only when her demeanour fits a very narrow ideal 'talkative and happy' on a regular basis (see also Webb, 1999). This is similar to a claim made by a participant in Goodley's study, that learning disabled people are expected by staff to act 'more normal than normal people' (Levine, cited in Goodley, 2001:215). Indeed, Sarah's concept of progression also involved unrealistic acceptance of the institutional regime. She also described the difficulties involved with expectations of progression:

Rebecca: And is there anything that you feel that you have to do to move on?
Sarah: Don't have any incidents.
Rebecca: What kind of incidents?
Sarah: Where you hit someone or be abusive to someone or get restrained.
Rebecca: And do you think you can manage that?
Sarah: Yes I've been managing it.
Rebecca: Is it hard?
Sarah: Yes it is sometimes when people wind you up.
Rebecca: What kind of things wind you up?

Sarah: Like I got hit last week off [names client] I got hit last week off her. And I just sat there and let her do it, I didn't want to hit back and that's why the staff said, 'That's good that you didn't hit back.' So that's why they're going to move me on.

(Interview, client, MSU)

Sarah's idea of progression was the absence of incidents, which aligns with the majority of staff's model. Worryingly, Sarah points out that she was expected to accept an assault and not retaliate, and that this was a sign to the staff that she was managing her anger. Staff member Wendy, however, did not see incidents as setbacks and acknowledged the role of staff in their onset.

Wendy: I think . . . that you've got to make some kind of a judgement and give them some kind of a chance and if you don't give them small goals then they're never going to go forward and they're never going to achieve what they want to do but [names client] she achieved a hell of a lot in her time down there, she did really well. She had a few incidents like, but that's what, I think you should do the goals, and you might have an incident but you've got to learn from that incident and think you might have to do it differently the next time and do it another way round. That's what they did and she achieved a lot really.

(Interview, unqualified staff, LSU)

Wendy advocates the use of 'small goals' to encourage progress, based on individual needs. She recognises that incidents may happen but that this is just part of the progress and that staff can avoid these by becoming more focussed on the reasons why the incident happened. This contradicts the idea that clients should learn to accept any sort of behaviour without retaliation, as in Sarah's comment. Wendy is articulating a way forward which is gradual and flexible, but which would involve adequate staffing and input.

Jane's situation involves self-monitoring and self-directing which was comprehended as progression. Jane was slowly given more trust by staff not to attempt suicide and this worked because she was supported through it and staff involvement was not significantly reduced at any point. This is a good example of where treatment and security can co-exist rather than being at odds with each other, as staff relinquished some of their control without traumatic consequences and Jane was seen to be self-directing eventually, despite this being referred to as 'taking control'. A more usual way of encouraging self-direction, however, was using the incentive system, which I will discuss next.

Incentive schemes: 'I wonder what they're going to give me'

One way behaviour was controlled and progress monitored for the women was by an incentive scheme, which was described by staff as individually designed around a person's perceived and documented risks. This was recorded by staff that had spent the most time with the person during the day. Some of the women might have received a 'cross' (X, or rather, not a 'tick') on their chart for refusing to go to work or for incidents of aggression. If no crosses were marked up for a certain period of time, the women were entitled to incentives such as 'pampering sessions' or visiting the nearest town. Incentives build up from ward-based activities to more substantial "rewards" such as trips to the cinema. Annie explained her incentives here:

Annie: Everyone's different. Like for me, I've got like an incentive chart. My incentive chart includes not being violent, no begging for treats.
Rebecca: No begging for treats?
Annie: Because I haven't got a lot of money sometimes [client] when she goes out she'll buy me stuff because she knows I haven't got the money to go out, but everybody blames it on me and says 'Well I've had to give it because Annie said she'd fall out with me' or, 'She wouldn't leave me alone until I give her it' kind of thing. Not begging for treats, attending work, no verbal outbursts, taking meds, and I think that's it. Oh and compliance with levels.
Rebecca: If you don't do those things . . .
Annie: You don't go the club and you don't get your incentive.
Rebecca: What's that?
Annie: Mine, the first one is pampering on the ward which I hardly ever get cos there's never enough staff and we can't have the stuff on the ward anyway because of [client who self-harms], second one if it hasn't changed is the canteen, the third one is [town], the fourth one is [larger town]. I did have weekly walks to [town] but I went once and that was it I didn't go after that and that were over 3 month ago. The very first week I did go I went with [staff] and I got some stuff out of the library and they've sent me about 4 letters now asking for them back but because no one's gone down I haven't been able to get them there, so I'll probably end up getting charged for them.

(Interview, client, LSU)

Annie previously was able to walk to the nearest town on a weekly basis, but then this became part of her incentive. It seems from her account that sometimes arrangements are changed and clients are required to be flexible if there is a lack of staff to take them. She talks about incentives as rewards for absence of certain undesirable behaviours such as violence, and flexibility in the form of acceptance of changes due to lack of staffing. It seems that for Annie, the incentive she expects is often not provided, yet she is encouraged to accept this and be flexible. I often noticed women planning ahead and anticipating trips and special occasions. Something out of the ordinary, like a birthday, was very much looked forward to. Occasionally staff did not seem to understand the importance of these events, and how disappointing it was to the clients when they were changed or cancelled.

Here, Ellie told me about her incentive arrangements:

Ellie: If I've achieved me stickers, then I can have my X-Box or my Nintendo DS.
Rebecca: And how do you get the stickers?

Ellie: By being good
Rebecca: And what does 'good' mean?
Ellie: Not hurting and not being abusive and that.

(Interview, client, LSU)

Ellie very clearly explained that she was rewarded for being 'good', which for her was the absence of abusive behaviour. On the MSU, however, the use of 'crosses' ensured that the focus remained on negative behaviours. Literature shows that 'bad' behaviour can be seen as a challenge to the rules rather than being understood in the context of an intolerable environment (Secker et al., 2004) and this can contribute to people staying in the system for longer. When rules are ambiguous, in other words people are not aware when they are breaking one, this can make it impossible to defend oneself or challenge the system (McCorkell, 2011). My fieldnotes show that staff are very much in charge of the incentives system and clients are not told formally that they have got a 'cross':

> There are lots of jokes about getting crosses when we go to the vending machine. The male staff is joking with the girls saying 'You've got sixteen crosses this week.' Just before the changeover, the staff are filling in sheets with ticks or crosses. There is one space for a.m. and one for p.m. The clients make efforts to try to see what is put down and mainly they can see.
>
> *(Fieldnotes, MSU)*

The clients did not find it easy to discuss or challenge their records, and it was clearly down to individual staff members whether the client was to have a cross or not that day. Brenda described how much power the staff have over the system here:

Brenda: To be honest, some of it is helpful for me because I know where I stand, but other times I think it's babyish because I think, 'I'll get a cross today.' And sometimes you're sitting there between six and eight and you're thinking "It's nearly eight o'clock, I wonder what they're going to give me?" Because I don't know what they're going to give me.

Brenda also points out that she thinks the system is 'babyish', like a star chart system designed for children, which uses a very basic behaviourist ideology (see also Flynn et al., 1997). Brenda goes on to say how clients might find out whether they have received a cross:

Brenda: We ask sometimes, sometimes they'll tell us, it depends what staff are on. Sometimes the staff come straight out and say "Oh yeah, you got a tick today", and other times they say "Oh no, you've got a cross and you've lost this, you've lost that, you've lost the other", but it all depends on how you've been. I've been all right for five days now.

(Interview, client, MSU)

Staff did not seem to be concerned about the childishness of the system; their conception of this system seemed to be that they were rewarding good behaviours rather than punishing bad behaviours:

Adele: And a lot of my involvement is in writing up guidelines for the staff to try and help them in how to interact with the women in all positive ways, to change behaviour from positive initiatives rather than taking things away from people. It's about a positive support for behavioural change rather than a negative, punitive approach, that's one of my key things.

(Interview, qualified staff)

Adele talked about how staff could 'change behaviour' by rewarding positively; she interpreted the incentives as providing extra rewards, rather than focussing on the crosses as Brenda mentioned. Stewart explained how he thought incentives can feed into overall concepts of progression:

Stewart: So if we can minimise those triggers, develop their coping strategies and – again – make them feel safe, then there become fewer and fewer reasons to have incidents. There are certain things, there's behavioural stuff that sounds a bit archaic I suppose, but they do work, it does tie in with real life, it is like the incentive programmes. If you're okay for a week then we'll do this as an extra thing, and it's important that we're not taking anything away if you don't do it, but if you can be okay, then we'll be able to do this. And again, we can do it from a clinical point; these are your risks, you score a five for this at the moment so if we can bring this down to three, we can take you to [larger town] on a one-to-one [one staff to accompany] rather than a two-to-one [two staff to accompany], or we can take you to the pictures when we don't think you're as risky in this kind of area.

(Interview, qualified staff)

Stewart also conceived the system as positively skewed. He described a system based on a reduction of risk due to feeling 'safe' and being 'okay' for a period of time. This is not how the clients saw the system, as they were focussing on 'crosses', which were given for many different reasons. For example, as Brenda pointed out here, sometimes work situations can be intolerable and leaving work results in a cross; Brenda had been telling me that a man was 'kicking off' at work and acting very disruptively. Brenda reported that she was the one who had to leave the situation and this resulted in her getting a cross, yet this was brushed off as unimportant by the staff:

Brenda: Say I went to work and there was somebody really bugging me and I said to them, "Look, I can't work with him", well then obviously they'd listen to the other person's side of things and then they'd take it on themselves to separate one of us and they'd say, "Come on Brenda, you've got to go back" and I'd say, "I don't want to go back. "Ah it's nothing, it's only a cross, never mind, you'll soon get over it." Why do I have to move when they started it? Why do I have to move, why do I have to go when he's started it?

(Interview, client, MSU)

Like Brenda, two other women referred to the system as childish:

Rebecca: So you don't agree with the incentive arrangement?
Helen: No, because it's kiddish, oh if you do this, and do this, you get this.
Rebecca: Do you not think it helps you to think about the future?
Helen: No, if you were 'on the out' you wouldn't have incentives.

(Interview, client, MSU)

Although Helen did see the incentive system as one based on reward rather than punishment, she was equating the use of incentives with incarceration, as she would not have incentives 'on the out'. When I asked Kate about incentives, she pointed out that she is not part of this system:

Kate: I don't need one [an incentive system]. They've said to me that I'm not that bad, I'm not bad enough, which is good cos I'm told I'm not bad enough to need one. So I must be getting better, so to me the fact that they've told me I'm not bad enough to need one makes me feel good.

(Interview, client, LSU)

Kate was happy that she did not have to work towards incentives which she equated with getting 'better'. This demonstrated the individualised nature of the system in place, but also poses the question of how Kate's progression is measured.

Incentives are used on the wards in order to get people to go to 'work' when they do not want to, and to encourage behavioural stability. It is interesting that women were required to be stable and predictable in their behaviour, yet were also required to understand when the schedules are changed unpredictably. When plans were changed by the service, even if these were part of incentives, the importance of these changes did not seem to be recognised by staff, and the anger of women was sometimes treated as irrational. Moreover, when women did manage to contain their feelings, this was not recognised within administrative processes which focussed on negative events.

I argue that the incentive system exemplifies the contradictions inherent in this type of service. Incentive systems are not peculiar to learning disability services but are a common method used to regulate behaviour in other total institutions (Holmes and Murray, 2012). The client has to negotiate a system which encourages 'playing the game' by signifying that the behaviour arises from personal will. The system retains control whilst at the same time demanding evidence of responsibility being taken however, sometimes this can result in resistance.

Resistance to progression: 'I played up on purpose'

As in other chapters, women were described by staff as 'needing' the institutional regime on some level, whether this was because they have not experienced the structure or boundaries in the past as in John's analysis, or because they lack confidence and skills to move out of a place of 'safety'. Staff sometimes talked about women sabotaging their progress by causing an incident just before they were due to move on, because they were afraid of the change:

Wendy: Well they don't like change do they? I've noticed that when they do come to move onto the next stage, that they will do something to destroy it because that's about their self-worth. . . . They're frightened, and probably [have] a lot of lack of confidence about moving on.

(Interview, staff, unqualified)

Aitken and Noble describe these acts of sabotage as women being accustomed to feeling hated, therefore negative power is the only power they are used to possessing (Aitken and Noble, 2001). This type of model implies that a way out of this cycle would be positive risk taking and sharing of power in positive ways. However, this needs to be carefully planned. Surrendering power too abruptly can cause people to lose confidence. As Wendy pointed out earlier, support for women can reduce as they are moved on and they are expected to be more independent. She considered that if the support continued longer, the women's moves would be more successful. In the MSU, support and reassurance offered by staff was considered by management to be superior to other parts of the service, yet this was not always talked about as a good thing. Some staff considered the women to be too happy or feel too safe to want to move on; Karen for example acknowledged the importance of built relationships and women's reluctance to leave them behind:

Karen: [Women are not progressing] because of the relationships, and they feel safe. I mean would you want to go out there really? I mean you're here, you've probably made the first friends you've ever made, the staff are kind to you, probably the first time ever anyone's been kind to them, they get their meals, they get nice things, incentives, probably go places they've never been to in their life. Why would you want to go?

Karen went on to say:

Karen: Um it's difficult because we have higher staffing ratios, um, they're kind of in this artificial bubble here where the staff are watching them, they can see them, they're very close to them, they feel very safe . . . And it's the trust and the relationships they make with the staff, they don't want to leave them, so you've got to have that balance.

(Interview, staff, qualified)

This type of situation must constitute a dilemma for staff: good staff/client relationships on one hand are discussed in positive terms, as keeping people safe, but on the other, as holding the client back and keeping them from moving on. Karen's interpretation was that the institutional regime and the therapeutic relationship is too successful and can cause problems, yet she was not acknowledging that the reason why it was a potential problem was because support drops drastically in the low secure areas due to there being fewer staff. Her solution to this reluctance to move on was to suggest making the MSU regime *more* restrictive and emphasise the independence women would experience after moving on:

Rebecca: So how do you prepare somebody for moving on then? What do you tell them? What do you do?

Karen: We would tell them that they will have far more opportunities on the low secure, they'll be able to go to work on their own, they'll have some free time. What we need to do as well here, there's some kind of business planning work to do on the MSU that makes it very specific how far, for instance if you're on the MSU you will only go to [Nearest town] or within a 5 mile radius, that kind of stuff. That needs to be done here, and then when they go to low secure there's much more incentive, you can go further afield, you can go on home visits, that kind of stuff. So the work still needs to be done to make this quite restrictive but not in a punitive way. Do you know what I mean? We need to make it more restrictive, they need to want to go to low secure: 'Bloody hell as soon as I get out I can go to there.' That's what we need to do and it is in the pipeline. We are trying to work on that.

(Interview, staff, qualified)

In my view, Karen's idea to place emphasis on independence and travelling further afield may work against progression, because it does not acknowledge the key issue, continued support. Karen's view of the MSU as discouraging progression was also a concern to a number of the qualified staff; however, the examples of women being seen as progressing and moving on that we have seen show that it is possible with the right amount of support throughout the process. Women clients talked about progression as a desirable thing. They did look forward to a future of moving on.

Any mention of sabotaging was discussed in purely strategic terms, for example Kate told me about 'playing up' so that she could move away from an unpleasant living situation after being moved to the step-down service.

Kate: [In the step-down service] There was a client there, it's not her fault it really isn't because she's, what do you call it, she can't, she doesn't have control over her bowels or her bladder. So she can't control them. But it always stunk of piss and shit, all over the place, all the time and we used to say to the staff 'Look, you need to do something with her because the thing is it's knocking us sick.' And they used to say, 'It doesn't concern you.' And I used to say 'Well actually it does because we're living like this.'

Rebecca: Yes course it does.

Kate: So I played up on purpose just to come back here.

Rebecca: Are you glad you're back [in the LSU]?

Kate: Yes.

(Interview, client, LSU)

Kate had made a decision to move back to the LSU and managed to bring this about, which would no doubt have implications on the length of her overall stay in the Service. Another of the women told me that she had moved back due to an incident of aggression that happened over Christmas which is a distressing time of the year for her:

> Katrina asks me if I want to see her bedroom. Whilst I am looking at her room I notice that her TV is smashed and taped over. Katrina sees me looking and begins to explain:
>
> *Katrina:*   Yes, I was living in [step-down service] but I had a bad time over Christmas so I had to come back. I wasn't well over Christmas.
>
> *Rebecca:*   Well, Christmas is a very stressful time for everyone I think.
>
> *Katrina:*   Well, there were things going on with my family and they came to visit, and then there were problems with staff – and I'm very sorry for what I did.
>
> *Me:*   It's OK, I understand.
>
> *Katrina:*   I'll be going back to the houses [step-down service] soon.
>
> *Staff:*   Yes well we're not sure about that at the moment.
>
> (Fieldnotes, LSU)

Katrina was disappointed that she had moved back to the LSU after making progress. Women were apparently moved backwards to a higher level of security for incidents of aggression, and this was construed as failure by some women. During my fieldwork, one of the women was being moved from the MSU to the LSU. She was extremely happy to be moving and considered it an achievement. There was renewed discussion about her future in light of the move and the other women on her flat participated in these discussions and congratulated her:

> Brenda tells me she is leaving to go to low secure. I ask her why and she tells me it is because someone else needs a place here. I ask if it has been acknowledged that her progression has been good and she said that someone had pointed this out. She was packing her stuff and was concerned that she had items put away in the loft and [staff member] comes in and says she needs someone to help her with the inventory. The other women are very happy for Brenda when they are told that she is moving on. They ask her if she needs help to pack her things and there are lots of questions. When Helen is

asking the staff member why she hasn't moved, he is very patient with her, saying that her behaviour has been 'impeccable' and that she will be able to move on when she's ready and it will happen. They discuss this at length and the staff member is extremely supportive and kind. Helen is worried that she will be in the MSU for years like Brenda. She says 'It's unsettling.'

(*Fieldnotes, MSU*)

It is evident that progression and moving on was important to the women and was seen as a positive step. Although, it is reported in the literature that some service users fear moving on due to the loss of safety and security of the locked ward (Parry-Crooke et al., 2000; Turton et al., 2011), these sentiments were not expressed by the women in my study.

Despite the organisational systems being construed by the women as restrictive, I did witness some women progressing during my fieldwork. They were gaining in confidence, engaging more with me and developing relationships with staff and clients. My fieldnotes here show that it is possible, although unusual, for women to progress reasonably quickly:

I see Ursula laughing and talking with the other women. She is keen to get involved in the activities and she looks bright and positive. When I think back to the first few times I met her, sitting on the sofa, staring into space and not engaging with anyone, seemingly shy and angry at the same time when I spoke to her, I cannot believe how far she has come in six months.

(*Fieldnotes, LSU*)

Unfortunately, I did not manage to talk to Ursula about her situation as she agreed to be observed but declined to be interviewed, although she was a striking example of how change can be possible.

Futures: 'Get my life back on track'

A sense of future was very important to the women in my study. Women in secure psychiatric services see the following attributes and support as important for their future: self-sufficiency, empowerment, life skills support and informal support networks (Richie, 2001; Parkes and Freshwater, 2012). These features were all expressed on some level by the women at Unit C. The women often talked about their futures; they did not want to stay in the service. Some discussed their future in terms of moving on *within* the service, to a less secure ward, and others talked about moving to other services. Those who mentioned moving out into the community were the largest group. They talked about 'getting out' and 'moving on'. Futures were generally discussed in terms of spending time with family members, for example:

Rebecca: What are you planning for your future? You've told me a little bit about moving to [home town].

Bonnie: Moving to a nice little supported living place. Meet up with my friends
            every now and then, go home meet and visit the family like my Dad,
            my Auntie. Yes.
Rebecca: Do you think you have to do anything to get to that point.
Bonnie: Just all my treatment. As I've said once my treatments over and done
            with then they'll look into how I am. My next CPA [Care Programme
            review meeting] will be in July.

(Interview, client, LSU)

Bonnie's plans involved complying with her treatment in order to have staff make positive judgements about her. As with other women, her statement did not convey any personal goals as a result of her stay, such as feeling more confident to move on. She did not say that *she* would judge how ready she was to move on, but the staff would do this. Bonnie had realistic ambitions for the future, supported living and seeing friends and family, reflecting her acceptance of the future in terms of disability, gender and social class. Brenda had similar aspirations:

Rebecca: And what do you see for your future when you've got out of here?
Brenda: I want to go into accommodation, sheltered accommodation or if not
            have me own flat, but with support workers. Like in [town], I had me
            own flat, but support workers used to come in daily just to give me
            medication then go home.

(Interview, client, MSU)

Like Brenda, most of the women expected that they would move to a supported living arrangement, and the majority talked about being able to have a job and see family and friends. Some of the younger women spoke about wanting to have children and had more normative expectations of the future that did not signify their label as a disabled woman:

Lorna: To get out and have some kids, get married, get my life back on track.
            I miss my family, miss my mates, miss drinking, miss having a laugh,
            going out on a Friday and Saturday night, having a laugh.

(Interview, client, MSU)

Marion's mother was elderly and in ill health when I spoke to her; Marion was extremely worried that something would happen to her mother whilst she was still at the unit. Marion's hopes for the future involved seeing her mother:

Marion: Folk have said I might be going to another unit somewhere else, but
            I'm hoping that if I do move somewhere else I'd be very close to my
            sister and my nephews and my niece and my brother in law.[2] But I do
            hope if I do move, sooner or later, that I'll be back before anything
            happens to my mum.

(Interview, client, LSU)

Some women gave very detailed plans for the future, for example Kate's plans included a future with her boyfriend. She was also realistic in assuming that they would need to live separately at first due to housing provision; learning disabled people usually cannot choose who they live with:

Kate: [Me and my boyfriend] we've talked about it a lot. We were saying that we're going to wait until we're both out, not one of us, both of us. Then we're going to go to, we're going to go abroad for a week or two, have a holiday and then we're just going to settle down, I'm going to have my flat, he's going to have his flat. But if that's going well after a couple of months still going well, then one of us will move in with the other one, which will be me because if it ever broke down I'd have somewhere to go, he wouldn't.

(Interview, client, LSU)

Many of the women spoke about wanting to work when they moved out, either in a paid job or volunteering, such as Reenie and Annie here:

Reenie: Well I'll try to get a little part-time job or sommat, in a cafe or sommat, washing up and cooking and, not a transport cafe, you know these little tea cafes.

(Interview, client, LSU)

Annie: I've always found that whenever I've got my head sorted out I'll always go back to a place where I can help people who are disabled or learning difficulties or whatever, but the main one after being in here is to look after and help people who self-harm, that's the main one that I want to do.

(Interview, client, LSU)

Employment often features in the literature on psychiatric recovery, with service users reporting that the working day provides them with confidence, structure and social integration (Ridgway, 2001; Provencher et al., 2002). Unfortunately, it would be quite difficult for some of the women in my study to gain the type of employment that they want when they move on, perhaps due to the nature of their offences which have brought them to Unit C, but also due to the lack of supported employment opportunities for learning disabled people in some areas. These plans for the future reflect the educational and cultural capital of the women, and they were realistic in terms of ambition.

These examples show the importance of family and friends to the women at Unit C. They also show how individual and personal people's futures are; thus a one-size-fits-all approach will not work. Crucially, the statements show that women are planning for the future and do not want to be detained long-term.

Conclusion

This chapter has shown that women's futures are not being adequately taken into account in the service. While clients had strong notions about their futures, staff priorities converged around day-to-day conflicts. It is crucial for staff and managers to keep in mind that the women have their futures to consider, which from their perspectives involve social integration, self-sufficiency and (re)building family relationships.

A main concept of progression discussed by participants was 'acceptance' – of other people's behaviour, and of the institutional regulations and routine, including last minute changes to this regime. Kate described that to move forward she has to make sure she does everything she is expected to do, such as go to work, take medication and carry on with therapy. Accepting other people, as in showing it was possible to be able to live together with other clients (as designated by staff) was also key. This I would argue further encourages passivity, in particular when women are expected to endure physical violence.

What is missing in these accounts of progression is what women wanted for themselves, in other words how they wanted their treatment to help them in their lives. In secure services literature, women report that they want: self-determination, empowerment, life skills support and informal support networks for the future (Richie, 2001; Parkes and Freshwater, 2012). Why are these criteria not used in concepts of progression with learning disabled women? Indeed the discourse of recovery did not feature on Unit C at all.

My research shows that personal notions of progression were missing in favour of 'proving' progression to staff in some way. Some of the women pointed out how difficult it was to show their progression. Tania clearly showed that to be considered 'happy' she had to act within very strict parameters, and Sarah said that she had to put up with physical assault without retaliation in order to show she was eligible to move on. This situation was exacerbated by the incentives system, which, although construed by staff as positive reinforcement, was seen as punitive and infantilising by clients. Hannah-Moffat (2000) refers to the 'neo-liberal strategies of responsibilizing' (2000:528), where women are 'empowered' to take responsibility for their actions, yet any failure to self-govern results in more punitive supervision, thereby '*re-enforcing* existing relations of power' (2000:529, emphasis added). I argue that this is the case here; the use of punishment negates any potential for empowerment and self-direction.

Both staff and clients attributed much of the progression that did occur on Unit C to individual care staff taking risks or making particular efforts to reach out for clients, which in the day-to-day running of the unit was quite difficult. Although staff mentioned that individual planning by the multidisciplinary team did include objectives for each client, this information was sometimes lost in the minutiae of daily incidents and control of the ward milieu. Focusing on clients' futures and progression involves communication between staff on the ground and those making the plans. It also involves time and sufficient staffing levels (Hatton and

Emerson, 1995), and for the organisation to recognise successful therapeutic relationships as important to progress. Disappointingly, these successful relationships were occasionally misconstrued by staff as preventing people from moving on because clients become reliant on them.

It can be argued that with adequate and sustained support, as Wendy and Jane show, it was possible for women to move on without substantial set-backs. Key to this, however, was a sense of trust within the framework of close therapeutic relationships. Some research found that treatment techniques try to steer women away from dependency and emotionality due to the idea that women's relational styles are deficient and irrational (McCorkel, 2003). It is considered possible to treat women as emotional and connected whilst supporting them to rehabilitate (McKim, 2008), but this is made much more difficult if relationships are construed as inherently problematic for clients.

Notes

1 Unconditional Positive Regard is a term coined by Carl Rogers (1951) and is still used in counselling and therapeutic discourse. It refers to positive treatment despite knowledge of the client's past and current issues.
2 Guidance indicates that people in residential services should be near to their families (Mansell, 1993), but many of my participants were far from their home town.

Bibliography

Adshead, G. (2011). Same but different: Constructions of female violence in forensic mental health. *International Journal of Feminist Approaches to Bioethics*, 4, 41–68.
Aitken, G., & Noble, K. (2001). Violence and violation: Women and secure settings. *Feminist Review*, 68, 68–88.
Aiyegbusi, A. (2002). Nursing interventions and future directions with women in secure services. *Forensic Focus*, 19, 136–150.
Alexander, R., Hiremath, A., Chester, V., Green, F., Gunaratna, I., & Hoare, S. (2011). Evaluation of treatment outcomes from a medium secure unit for people with intellectual disability. *Advances in Mental Health and Intellectual Disabilities*, 5, 22–32.
Barron, P., Hassiotis, A., & Banes, J. (2002). Offenders with intellectual disability: The size of the problem and therapeutic outcomes. *Journal of Intellectual Disability Research*, 46, 454–463.
Beresford, P. (2005). Social work and a social model of madness and distress. *Social Work and Social Sciences Review*, 12, 59–73.
Brackenridge, I., & Morrissey, C. (2010). Trauma and post-traumatic stress disorder (PTSD) in a high secure forensic learning disability population: Future directions for practice. *Advances in Mental Health and Intellectual Disabilities*, 4, 49–56.
Flynn, M., Griffiths, S., Byrne, L., & Hynes, K. (1997). "I'm stuck here with my poxy star chart": Listening to mentally disordered offenders with learning disabilities. In P. Ramcharan, G. Roberts, G. Grant & J. Borland (Eds.), *Empowerment in everyday life* (pp. 143–155). London: Jessica Kingsley.
Goodley, D. (2001). Learning difficulties, the social model of disability and impairment: Challenging epistemologies. *Disability & Society*, 16, 207–231.

Hannah-Moffat, K. (2000). Prisons that empower. *British Journal of Criminology*, 40, 510–531.

Hatton, C., & Emerson, E. (1995). Staff in services for people with learning disabilities: An overview of current issues. *Mental Handicap Research*, 8, 215–219.

Holland, A., & Meddis, R. (1993). People living in community homes: The influences on their activities. *Mental Handicap Research*, 6, 333–345.

Holmes, D., & Murray, S. J. (2012). A critical reflection on the use of behaviour modification programmes in forensic psychiatry settings. In D. Holmes, T. Rudge & A. Perron (Eds.), *(Re) thinking violence in health care settings: A critical approach* (pp. 21–30). Farnham: Ashgate.

Mancini, A. D. (2008). Self-determination theory: A framework for the recovery paradigm. *Advances in Psychiatric Treatment*, 14, 358–365.

Mansell, J. (1993). *Services for people with learning disabilities and challenging behaviour or mental health needs: Report of a project group.* London: HMSO.

Mansell, J., Beadle-Brown, J., Skidmore, C., Whelton, B., & Hutchinson, A. (2006). People with learning disabilities in "out-of-area" residential placements: 1: Policy context. *Journal of Intellectual Disability Research*, 50, 837–844.

Mccorkel, J. A. (2003). Embodied surveillance and the gendering of punishment. *Journal of Contemporary Ethnography*, 32, 41–76.

Mccorkell, A. D. (2011). *Am I there yet? The views of people with learning disability on forensic community rehabilitation.* D.Clin.Psych. Thesis, University of Edinburgh.

Mckim, A. (2008). "Getting gut-level" punishment, gender, and therapeutic governance. *Gender & Society*, 22, 303–323.

Mcwade, B. (2014). *Recovery in an "arts for mental health" Unit.* Ph.D. Thesis, Lancaster University.

Parkes, J., & Freshwater, D. (2012). The journey from despair to hope: An exploration of the phenomenon of psychological distress in women residing in British secure mental health services. *Journal of Psychiatric and Mental Health Nursing*, 19, 618–628.

Parry-Crooke, G., Oliver, C., & Newton, J. (2000). *Good girls: Surviving the secure system, a consultation with women in high and medium secure psychiatric settings.* London: Women in Special Hospitals (WISH).

Pollack, S. (2007). "I'm just not good in relationships" victimization discourses and the gendered regulation of criminalized women. *Feminist Criminology*, 2, 158–174.

Provencher, H. L., Gregg, R., Mead, S., & Mueser, K. T. (2002). The role of work in the recovery of persons with psychiatric disabilities. *Psychiatric Rehabilitation Journal*, 26, 132–144.

Resnick, S. G., Fontana, A., Lehman, A. F., & Rosenheck, R. A. (2005). An empirical conceptualization of the recovery orientation. *Schizophrenia Research*, 75, 119–128.

Richie, B. E. (2001). Challenges incarcerated women face as they return to their communities: Findings from life history interviews. *Crime & Delinquency*, 47, 368–389.

Ridgway, P. (2001). Restorying psychiatric disability: Learning from first person recovery narratives. *Psychiatric Rehabilitation Journal*, 24, 335.

Rogers, C. R. (1951). *Client-centered therapy: Its current practice, implications, and theory.* London: Constable.

Rossiter, K. R. (2012). *Victimization, trauma, and mental health: Women's recovery at the interface of the criminal justice and mental health systems.* Ph.D. Thesis, Simon Fraser University.

Schrank, B., & Slade, M. (2007). Recovery in psychiatry. *Psychiatric Bulletin*, 31, 321–325.

Secker, J., Benson, A., Balfe, E., Lipsedge, M., Robinson, S., & Walker, J. (2004). Understanding the social context of violent and aggressive incidents on an inpatient unit. *Journal of Psychiatric and Mental Health Nursing*, 11, 172–178.

Simpson, A. I., & Penney, S. R. (2011). The recovery paradigm in forensic mental health services. *Criminal Behaviour and Mental Health*, 21, 299–306.

Travers, R. (2013). *Treatment of women in forensic settings: Women and psychiatric treatment: A comprehensive text and practical guide*. London: Routledge.

Turton, P., Demetriou, A., Boland, W., Gillard, S., Kavuma, M., Mezey, G. . . . Zadeh, E. (2011). One size fits all: Or horses for courses? Recovery-based care in specialist mental health services. *Social Psychiatry and Psychiatric Epidemiology*, 46, 127–136.

Vaughan, P. (2003). Secure care and treatment needs of individuals with learning disability and severe challenging behaviour. *British Journal of Learning Disabilities*, 31, 113–117.

Ward, T., & Brown, M. (2004). The good lives model and conceptual issues in offender rehabilitation. *Psychology, Crime & Law*, 10, 243–257.

Webb, T. (1999). Voices of people with learning difficulties. In J. Swain & S. French (Eds.), *Therapy and learning difficulties: Advocacy, participation and partnership* (pp. 47–71). Oxford: Butterworth Heinemann.

Yacoub, E., Hall, I., & Bernall, J. (2008). Secure in-patient services for people with learning disability: Is the market serving the user well? *Psychiatric Bulletin*, 32, 205–207.

7   Intersections
Making conclusions

I set out on this research to explore people's experiences of living and working on a locked learning disability unit. When I embarked on this project, I was aware of the body of ethnographic research set in mental health residential settings, including those categorised as 'forensic'. Whilst not trying to replicate this work, and acknowledging its relevance to the women in my study, I hope my work highlights the importance of researching the features and particularities of services specifically for people diagnosed as learning disabled. This book adds to existing scholarship in gender and disability, but is situated within a setting which has so far been overlooked by ethnographic researchers.

My research questions were: How do clients and staff experience day-to-day life here? How do women feel they are able to progress through the service? How do experiences of coercive management affect this progression? During my research, these questions evolved into more conceptual ones, such as: How do interpretations of gender and disability influence staff and clients' experiences on the unit? How do the discourse and the practices within the unit shape ideas about gender and disability? In seeking to answer these questions, I have shown that gender and disability cannot be disentangled from women's experiences and the accounts that are used to understand them.

In endeavouring to answer the original research questions, I found that ideas and expectations about women, their impairments and their social class were woven within the fabric of the institution and made their marks on day-to-day experiences; an example of this were the activities offered to women during the day and evening. Although the 'menu' of activities seemed to be quite diverse, some women did not have a choice of all of these activities and, especially those living on the MSU, were allocated quite risk-averse ones. 'Pamper' sessions and 'colouring in' reflect the gendered nature of these activities, and the expectations that *learning disabled* women will find these things relaxing. On a positive note, the Women's Action Group was considered a progressive step towards client involvement in the service, and the events organised by the members were encouraging and inclusive, taking into account clients' suggestions and recommendations. Nevertheless, not all women had access to this group. Whilst I was completing my fieldwork, the organisation was implementing person-centred Occupational Therapy which the clients and staff were anticipating. I hope that this development addresses the issues I have described here.

In exploring ideas about how women progress through the service, I found myself asking what the purpose of the service was. In formal descriptions, the service is described as providing 'treatment' and 'rehabilitation', yet these descriptions are only meaningful if the objectives filter into day-to-day life. In my observations and interviews, talk about behavioural stability pervaded concepts of progress to the cost of ideas of personal recovery, or treatment and rehabilitation. Perhaps this is how rehabilitation is conceived at Unit C. It was clear that women were accessing psychological therapy, yet support staff were not trained in counselling, sometimes leaving women at a loose end when returning from a therapy session, as described in Chapter 5. Although I have criticised the focus on women's pasts at the expense of talk about their futures, women's experiences of abuse and violence are extremely important when it comes to therapy and treatment. As I have argued, the consequences of these events can be taken into account as long as women's strengths and future aspirations also feature in the conversation.

The social history relating to women's admittance to and management in these services in Britain cannot be denied; there are many stories of learning disabled women who were incarcerated against their will and who lived all of their lives within the asylum. I have shown that some aspects of this history are still evident today within such regulatory practices as exclusion from the home community and segregation of men and women within the institution. Yet at the same time contemporary policy has taken an opposing position, promoting the ideals of 'choice' and 'control' and 'independence'. This incompatibility between policy and practice is most evident when it comes to the management measures used to keep women in line, increasing dependence, whilst expectations within local and national policy are that clients are responsible and self-reliant.

This is what McWade portrays so well when she describes how the 'shame of the asylum years where patients were often incarcerated for life now manifests itself in a fear of, or aversion to, patient dependency on services' (McWade, 2014:182). Staff in McWade's study of an 'arts for mental health' unit seemed to think of dependency in terms of the harmful history of institutionalisation, and these aversions to dependency, she argues, are strengthened by the current neoliberal political discourse around the self-responsible individual which permeates media and policy. This discourse was evident in my interviews with staff; there were worries about clients becoming reliant on coercive methods such as seclusion, as well as concerns about them becoming too comfortable in the service and enjoying their relationships with staff too much. Yet I have argued that these feelings of safety can contribute to progression as long as steps are taken gradually. Another concern related to this was the restricted connections with the local community and links with family and friends, bringing to mind Goffman's Total Institution model of segregation from society. I argue that dependency on the service would be less of a concern for staff if access to the outside world was more plentiful.

Accepting that the present study cannot be separated from the history of institutionalisation is key in my argument, and using these themes in tandem with gender and disability studies, I aim to now explore the conceptual questions which arose during my study. Finally, I will use these to formulate some recommendations for change.

Intersections

Women with disabilities have been exposed to many and varying experiences of oppression and discrimination (Thomas, 2006), and there are often well-meaning motivations behind injustices that they experience (Young, 2009). As I described in Chapter 1, the clients in my study may be subjected to certain experiences in society because they are situated at the intersection of disability, gender and social class, and particular to this study, these categorisations also feature judgements about behaviour which deviates from the norm or is criminalised. In this section, I will look at how women's experiences relate to intersectionality (Crenshaw, 1991), which can be described as the analysis of the relationship between different categories of identity. Theories of intersectionality explore inequalities by focussing on the interplay between different sources of oppression (Mattsson, 2014) and I shall describe a few examples of this interplay on Unit C here. As in other literature (Adshead, 2000; Vaughn and Stamp, 2003; McWade, 2014), I noticed some paradoxes or contradictions evident in the practices and discourse. I will use these contradictions to illustrate the tensions inherent in this type of service and to form my reflections.

Disability was manifested on Unit C in the power disparity between staff and clients which was evident in many areas of life, for example the admittance process, where many women had not been told they would be staying at the unit and the fact that they are not given a release date. Also, ideas about disability were expressed in concepts of progression which always involved staff's judgements rather than personally determined outcomes; herein the dominance of services over people was unmistakeable. The presumption of incompetence is inherent in society's notions of learning disabilities, which provides justification for professionals making decisions on behalf of people. This in turn influences the continuation of dependency.

The staff noticed this issue of power imbalance, the difficulty of maintaining an equilibrium between therapy and control featured in their interviews. They talked about power differentials and how they cause conflict, which in turn brings about coercive practices. For example, when Iona observed in Chapter 4, '*They get you to do things either by being really nice or really horrible. But do you not think that's because of the way we set our role up? . . . because we're the jailors.*' However, this tension did not seem to be tackled at management level, for example by encouraging partnership-type relationships, or a working alliance. Indeed, positive relationships between staff and clients were sometimes described as fostering women's dependence on the service, and staff were under pressure to withhold their support at key moments such as during seclusion to prevent 'reinforcement' – as described in Chapter 5 by Adele. I have argued that the practice of withholding support illuminates these power relationships further and substantiates the view that learning disabled people require control. Phillips discusses the reasons for this control when she refers to how the 'perceived incompetence of the *mind* is then transported to a perceived incompetence of the *body*. Hence a situation is created where the body has to be controlled, cared for and regulated' (Phillips, 2007:507, emphasis in original). Often, this situation is created with good intentions, as learning disabled people are considered to need protection and guidance (Lövgren and Bertilsdotter Rosqvist, 2014).

This notion of protection was evident on Unit C, particularly around the regulation of relationships. There was a lack of clear information about sexual relationships and a need for some sort of sexual awareness education to encourage self-determination in relationships. Ideas about gender and disability were markedly evident in notions of vulnerability and protection where sexual relationships were involved. I have argued that this regulation is rationalised in terms of women's vulnerability stemming from their past experiences rather than directly related to the male clients' presence on the unit as should have been the case. As others have argued, learning disabled women have often been described in the contradictory depictions of vulnerability and dangerousness (Williams, 1992; Phillips, 2007), both of which necessitate the use of management and protection. However, when protection becomes limiting, this is when power struggles and resistance can ensue.

My argument is not that individual staff bring about this power disparity; power was not unidirectional on Unit C, and staff and clients did share some experiences. For example in Chapter 4, I described how staff were subjected to various forms of regulation from management and other staff in terms of their relationships with clients. Furthermore, staff had to deal with retaliation from women as a result of resistance to the restrictions of life on the Unit. In this sense, staff were situated between two conflicting expectations. They were operating within a discourse of control which did not accept resistance as legitimate and this caused various tensions. I think these tensions contributed to the ambiguous views of relationships on the unit: relationships as supportive on one hand but also constraining on the other. This was related to women's learning disability status in terms of policy – for example current learning disability policy and its objective of independence - but also their gender in the way women were judged on their (in)ability to maintain successful relationships throughout their lives. Difficult relationships were particularly discussed in terms of gender, with women being described yet again in contradictory terms, as lacking in relational skills on one hand, as well as being clever and expert manipulators on the other.

Gender was especially marked out in staff descriptions of women as exceptionally problematic to work with. This was expressed in judgements made by staff about aggression, in particular ideas about women's tendency towards relational aggression, and how much more difficult it is to deal with than overt aggression. The constitution of women clients as problematic on the Unit sets them apart from staff, 'othering' them, which in turn creates conflict and causes expressions of distress. Staff find these expressions extremely difficult and feel that they have no choice but to use coercive methods to deal with them. This could be described as using physical security in place of relational security (Department of Health,

2010), where women are encouraged to be passive and compliant in order to show progression. I suggest that this is a consequence of expectations of femininity and what is 'acceptable' in terms of anger shown by women. I have argued that difficult behaviour can be seen as communication of distress or fear, that women should be provided with a 'safe space' to be angry, and I maintain that emphasis should be placed on resolving conflict, allowing people to learn valuable skills from this process

As I have mentioned earlier in this chapter, staff interpretation of women's past trauma could often put them at a disadvantage. Some of the women described their past experiences to me and they were often horrific and undeniably caused them distress. When described by staff, women's pasts were conceived in terms of bad role models, chaotic lifestyles and lack of structure and discipline. It could be argued that social and economic deprivation contributed to these interpretations, as disabled people frequently experience poverty as a consequence of discrimi-nation (Shakespeare, 1994; Björnsdóttir and Traustadóttir, 2010) and learning disabled people are more likely to experience adverse life events compounded by poverty (Hatton and Emerson, 2004). Knowledge of this inequality may cause staff to make assumptions based on the social class of clients and what is appro-priate for them, for example in terms of what clients were offered for 'treats' and trips out, and were replicated in women's own plans for their future lives in the community.

I suggest that a process of gendering is also taking place here. For example, Chapter 4 showed how women were often described as victims, and this con-veyed ideas of lasting damage that caused women to be in danger of replaying the past. Although these notions of women's experiences were productive in some respects, specifically in providing reasons for their current distress, I argue that perception of pasts as permanently damaging precluded a focus on *futures*. This in turn left very little space for attention to aspirations and goals on a day-to-day basis as evidenced by women's understandings of progression. There was sparse talk about personal goals, with intentions of compliance to treatment and work routines taking precedence. This focus on work could be attributed to traditional notions of work as 'cure' (see McWade, 2014) or the contribution of a structured day-to-day rehabilitation (Bose, 2009). However, as I have mentioned, there was a tension between personal and organisational definitions of progression. Progres-sion in Unit C was usually interpreted in terms of behavioural stability; however, my claim is that personal aspirations for the future are key to progression. In agreement with McCorkell (2011:115), I argue that women should have

> clear care pathways which outline the individual goals and time frames for gradual progression . . . This is to make clear what is required of the indi-vidual in order to progress as well as how to achieve this, but also to make this a tangible reality, enhancing hope for the future.

Another contradiction I was made aware of was the tension between treat-ment and coercion. Many of the staff were concerned about their conflicting roles and requirements, in particular the balance between control and therapy (also described by Bowers, 2006). They found it difficult to embody both therapist and jailor. Some authors assert that treatment and security should be construed as requirements of each other in order to promote recovery and progression (Pouncey and Lukens, 2010; Simpson and Penney, 2011), and when individual needs and futures are taken into account, I suggest this can be possible. For Travers, the aim of a forensic service for women should be to 'maximise the empowerment process, whilst allowing [the woman] to acknowledge and accept her own responsibility and accountability for both her behaviours and their consequences' (Travers, 2013:81). This can only happen, in my view, if there is recognition of the value of supportive relationships at an organisational level, and a two-way process of communication, where women's behavioural responses are considered in terms of the contexts and preceding events. Success in future community integration and accessing community resources can be dependent on the nature and quality of relationships with others. Therefore, although aspirations of independence are reflected in policy documents such as *Valuing People* (Department of Health, 2001), *inter*dependence should be key (Carnaby, 1998; Reindal, 1999).

Linking with this issue is a further contradiction, the discrepancy between positive risk taking and coercion. Service aims as reflected in discourse and terminology include fostering autonomy in people, which inherently involves allowing them to take risks. Yet, women view the visible and omnipresent coercive techniques of constant observation, physical intervention and seclusion as controlling and sometimes punitive, encouraging compliance and passivity. The competing aims of dependence and autonomy here mean that women find it difficult to deduce what is expected of them in terms of behaviour and how to demonstrate that they are progressing.

In agreement with Phillips (2007), women's bodies on Unit C were indeed sites of regulation and control, evidenced within discourse as well as action. I argue that as a matter of urgency, the organisation needs to deal with the way women clients are understood throughout the staff groups, as Adele described:

Adele: It's a shame really that women have a reputation, so as soon as you say to somebody, 'You'll be working with the women', It's like, 'Oh no, they're hard work aren't they?' And that seems to be a reputation that's there, and is into the culture of the place before people have ever had the experience of knowing whether they're hard work or not.

(Interview, qualified staff)

Adele's quote illustrates perfectly the problematic essentialist preconceptions around women that I have shown in this work. One way to transform this would be to increase the involvement of women clients in staff training, so that staff are able to learn about women and their experiences and aspirations, within an alternative power dynamic. I argue that if the discourse around women on Unit C were to change, and staff were offered support to enable this to happen, a more positive culture among all in the women's service may result. In particular I feel that if staff were given training and guidance about the social model of disability and the ways in which impairments can be brought about and exacerbated by socially imposed barriers, this may encourage a shift in culture.

Morgan (2012) recommends that the social model of disability should be taken on board as a 'threshold concept', a concept which disrupts traditional ways of thinking and cultivates a new ideology. This insight may encourage staff to think about making positive adjustments to the service women receive, rather than focussing on the imbalance that women are perceived to bring about, and it would be one idea for a positive outcome from this work.

In relation to women and the essentialist discourse which proliferates throughout the Service, I would argue for the adoption of a *performative* concept of gender (Butler, 1990), where gender is seen as continuously socially enacted or performed. Femininity therefore, is understood as a performance but also formative, in that it reproduces ideas of a 'natural' way of being in the world. Taking this on board at Unit C as a further 'threshold concept' would challenge notions of deviance as biological and pathological, and instead women's behaviour would be recognised as socially established, relational and contextual.

My research has shown the contextual contingence and socially constituted nature of what is classed as 'difficult' behaviour, in particular demonstrating how supportive relationships could transform this behaviour. There was no suggestion that the behavioural incentive systems caused any similar results, indicating that these schemes should be seriously re-evaluated. I hope too, that my research will be taken on board by Unit C as a constructive and faithful reflection of the setting as it was when I did my fieldwork.

I disseminated my work accessibly to all staff and clients at Unit C, and I will detail my recommendations for policy and practice at the end of this chapter. First, however, I would like to share some reflections about my study which may help other researchers who are considering embarking on a similar project.

Reflections

I feel that the use of ethnography greatly benefitted my project and I would recommend its use for work with marginalised groups in any setting. It allowed me to get to know staff and clients and explain the research to them, ensuring ethical adherence. Ethnography is not an easy methodology to implement, there were many times when I felt sad, worried and distressed, and although there were some other difficulties associated with the use of observation as I will explain, I feel the quality of data emerged directly as a result of my choice of method.

The difficulties I encountered were mainly associated with the length of time it took to gain consent, explaining the research and the reason for such a broad remit (in response to being asked, 'What is your hypothesis?') As I have mentioned previously, when I was embarking on my research fieldwork, the BBC televised a Panorama undercover report detailing footage of shocking abuse and brutality which took place in a private learning disability unit (Chapman, 2011). In response to this report, Unit C held a number of meetings to discuss lessons learned from the programme. Staff were made acutely aware of safeguarding issues and I feel they were worried that I might have been critically observing their actions; some staff appeared suspicious of my presence on the wards and one staff member withdrew her consent during this time. Nevertheless, on the whole both staff and clients were very welcoming and open despite the interruption in their routine that I may have caused.

I feel that the observation allowed me to see people in the context of their daily lives, interacting and supporting each other. Goodley and Rapley's (2001) article looking at self-advocacy groups argues that investigating the lived experience of learning disabled people can enable the 're-socializing of impairment' (2001:231). They discuss how assumptions of incapability can be disrupted by instances of resistance which situate the person in 'relational understandings' (2001:231), in other words looking at how people manage to get by, despite the dominant way of thinking which naturalises and individualises impairment. I think my work exemplifies this idea, by showing how women retain their sense of self despite significant regulation.

Ethnography allowed me to comment on silences and absences, which would not have been possible using an interview method. Despite entering the field with few expectations, in my fieldwork I noticed a lack of discussion around fundamental topics such as sexuality and family links which may reflect an adherence to confidentiality, or may indicate that these are not being dealt with. So although I cannot make specific claims about these absences, I was a able to flag them up to the organisation as issues which may need addressing.

Along with silences and absences, I saw many instances where good practice prevailed, such as the consideration and energy that many staff put into their work, and the warmth evident in many relationships, both between the women and with staff. Again, such issues may not have been illuminated during an interview-based study. This made me realise that even though these women are detained in a very restrictive environment, there are still moments of pleasure and kindness and even joy. This, combined with the personalities and charisma of many of the clients and staff, ensured that the experience of spending time on Unit C will stay with me throughout my life.

Recommendations

Staff and clients had a lot to say about the service. Both groups of people had understandings about what was and was not working, yet had very little scope to change the status quo. In this section I will bring together some reflections about how to address the issues I have described, some of which I gleaned from people's accounts, and also some of my own which I have ascertained during my research. To build on this section, I suggest that there should be a forum where both groups are formally able to put forward their ideas for a better future and where this will be taken seriously and acted upon.

At policy level, I suggest that community services should offer more support to learning disabled people and their families, as they are at risk of experiencing structural inequality and discrimination. Learning disabled girls and women should not be excluded from sex education, and any allegations of abuse should not be ignored or disbelieved. Indeed, any education which encourages self-determination and assertiveness should be welcomed. People with learning disabilities should be offered more support at times of transition from child to adult services, to avoid them experiencing a period of uncertainty. I further suggest that the procedure and rationale for admittance to secure units for people with learning disabilities should be investigated and formalised – it seems that the policy aims of providing 'choice' and 'control' are only applicable to certain groups of people.

Ryan and Julian (2015) insist that the system of detaining people for reasons of challenging behaviour is flawed, and that the service provision is unacceptable and inappropriate. In terms of learning disabled offenders, it has been recommended numerous times that small, therapeutic community units are more suitable for this group, in particular women, yet large secure units with a more correctional ethos remain. A concerning implication of this is that people are being detained miles from their home town, sometimes for many years. Treatment programmes should have clearly defined goals and end dates and be designed in consultation with the clients and families (Hatton, 2014). As I have shown, power relations between staff and clients should also be contemplated at policy level, which would entail acknowledgement of the coercive methods used with learning disabled people and the value of finding therapeutic alternatives. The fundamental importance of supporting positive relationships should underpin all policy developments.

For individual services, I have further recommendations.

All of my suggestions call for more proactive engagement with the women. In the face of conflict for example, services should be allowing for time to discuss the reasons for women's anger, rather than using more restrictive measures. Acknowledgement, rather than repression of anger needs to take place, and the connection between powerlessness and anger needs to be recognised. Anger is being seen as pathological, yet there should be a shared awareness that frustration arising from incarceration and its regulations can cause people to be angry. As a way forward, it would help if anger was seen as communication, and utilised as a way to address issues that are under the surface. Opportunities for resolving disputes should not be missed. Everyone should be able to benefit from debriefing following an incident, and separate spaces for expressions of anger should be available. I argue that this would allow greater understanding and expression and reduce the amount of longer-term relational aggression which staff find so wearing. Of course, this would necessitate more staff to be available on a daily basis, but perhaps would reduce the amount of staff having to be available for emergency situations such as seclusion.

My research also calls for a greater focus on relationships and how to successfully negotiate them. There should be recognition of the value of supportive relationships at the policy and organisational level, and a two-way process of communication, where women's behavioural responses are considered in terms of the contexts and preceding events. Success in future community integration and accessing community resources can be dependent on the nature and quality of relationships with others; therefore, the service should acknowledge that people need to forge relationships of their own choosing. Furthermore, staff need to accept that things will sometimes go wrong and that women will need extra support at these times, and these experiences will add to their relational skills.

In particular, concerning relationships, it is extremely important that links to the people's 'outside' life are kept active. Those family members and friends with whom women had supportive relationships prior to admittance should be encouraged to have more involvement in their lives. The lack of discussion around family and important people on the wards may have been due to concerns about confidentiality; yet, some women did mention that they would like more contact with their family. It is clear from my participants that some people are placed in these services far from home and stay for many years; therefore the value of maintaining positive family/friend links is vital for future support when moving on. This needs to be reflected in policy and practice throughout the service. Although it is understandable that staff in my research did regard some families as problematic, as one of their informal roles seemed to be protecting the women from negative family relationships, it is important that staff consider families and friends where appropriate, in more positive ways rather than something from which to protect people.

Although Unit C is introducing new therapies for those diagnosed with BPD, I would suggest that any training for staff should focus on understandings of how 'manipulative' behaviour comes about, as a way of obtaining crucial attention in a very controlling environment. I would suggest teaching staff to consider behaviour using external and contextual criteria, rather than seeing the issue as internal and as part of the woman. Further developing staff understanding of attachment theory and developmental trauma may help with this.

Issues about vulnerability in relation to sexual relationships were directly linked to the presence of male offenders in the service and this influenced the prevailing discourse. Ideally on Unit C, the women's MSU service should be removed from the area which includes the men's wards. Services should consider allowing intimate and sexual relationships and recognise the benefits these can bring to people's lives.

If it is unrealistic to enable women to experience sexual relationships in this setting where they may reside for a large part of their lives, then clear policies and procedures informed by service users must be introduced which have the scope to be individualised. Further research might focus on the development of these policies which should be designed in collaboration with women and communicated openly to them. It is crucial to use this strategy to develop education programmes which promote self-determination in order to allow people to make informed choices about relationships in the future. Furthermore, sexuality needs to be more broadly conceived, incorporating knowledge about masturbation and romance for example.

Discussions about futures should not be overshadowed by ideas about women's pasts. Objectives should include acknowledging people's strengths and future aspirations, including positive risk taking. Any discussions about progression should include looking to future competencies, rather than largely dealing with current issues. Crucially, women should be encouraged to consider and articulate personal outcomes that they would like the service to fulfil. Staff/client relationships cannot be disentangled from concepts of progression, and these need to be consolidated before gradual autonomy is introduced.

Incentive systems in services should be reconsidered along with the behaviour management options available. Despite the intended objective of positive reinforcement, both practices are seen by clients to be punitive. Unit C needs to find other ways to deal with disruptive behaviour, some of which I have already mentioned such as allowing some demonstration of anger, but also avoiding placing women in seclusion as soon as they arrive. This is linked to information provision as well. If women are not given information about their stay and what to expect, they feel bewildered and distressed right from the start.

Confidential forums for staff discussion would be beneficial, where staff are able to challenge and reassure each other. A place to discuss incidents and relationships, offer advice and vent frustration should be provided. This may support staff to work better with the women with whom they experience conflict. Further, staff training should be enhanced. Introducing the concept of the social model of disability into staff training will encourage the staff focus to relocate from clients' deficits to service deficits, and Unit C will become more person-centred. The involvement of clients in staff training should be extended, to allow a forum where clients are outside the power differential, to impart knowledge of 'how it feels' to live in Unit C.

Of course, these recommendations are dealing with the day-to-day minutiae of life on such units. An overarching recommendation would be to question the purpose of these units, whether they are successfully offering treatment and care, or mainly serving to confine people. I suggest that the wealth of staff expertise and knowledge in such units should be used productively to offer individualised treatment and support that involves the family and friends of the person. Further, this knowledge and understanding could be harnessed to provide families with support and information at an earlier point, before crisis strategies and inpatient care are needed. By viewing disability and gender as part of a bigger picture, at a societal as well as an individual level, policymakers and individual services could make this change.

Bibliography

Adshead, G. (2000). Care or custody? Ethical dilemmas in forensic psychiatry. *Journal of Medical Ethics*, 26, 302–304.

Björnsdóttir, K., & Traustadóttir, R. (2010). Stuck in the land of disability? The intersection of learning difficulties, class, gender and religion. *Disability & Society*, 25, 49–62.

Bose, S. (2009). Containment and the structured day. In J. Clarke-Moore & A. Aiyegbusi (Eds.), *Therapeutic relationships with offenders: An introduction to the psychodynamics of mental health nursing* (pp. 105–119). London: Jessica Kingsley Publishers.

Bowers, L. (2006). On conflict, containment and the relationship between them. *Nursing Inquiry*, 13(3), 172–180.

Butler, J. (1990). Gender trouble, feminist theory, and psychoanalytic discourse. In L. Nicholson (Ed.), *Feminism/postmodernism* (pp. 324–340). New York: Routledge.

Carnaby, S. (1998). Reflections on social integration for people with intellectual disability: Does interdependence have a role? *Journal of Intellectual and Developmental Disability*, 23, 219–228.

Chapman, M. (2011). Undercover care: The abuse exposed. *BBC Panorama*.

Crenshaw, K. (1991). Mapping the margins: Intersectionality, identity politics, and violence against women of color. *Stanford Law Review*, 43(6), 1241–1299.

Department of Health. (2001). *Valuing people: A new strategy for learning disability for the 21st century*. London: Department of Health.

Department of Health. (2010). *See, think, act: Your guide to relational security*. London: Department of Health.

Goodley, D., & Rapley, M. (2001). How do you understand "learning difficulties"? Towards a social theory of impairment. *Mental Retardation*, 39, 229–232.

Hatton, C. (2014). *The times, they are (not) changing*. Available at http://chrishatton.blogs pot.co.uk/2014/11/the-times-they-are-not-changing.html (Accessed 26/11/2014).

Hatton, C., & Emerson, E. (2004). The relationship between life events and psychopathology amongst children with intellectual disabilities. *Journal of Applied Research in Intellectual Disabilities*, 17, 109–117.

Lövgren, V., & Bertilsdotter Rosqvist, H. (2014). "More time for what?" Exploring intersecting notions of gender, work, age and leisure time among people with cognitive disabilities. *International Journal of Social Welfare*, Early Online Version, Available at http://onlinelibrary.wiley.com/journal/10.1111/(ISSN)1468-2397/earlyview (Accessed 01/2015).

Mattsson, T. (2014). Intersectionality as a useful tool anti-oppressive social work and critical reflection. *Affilia*, 29, 8–17.

Mccorkell, A. D. (2011). *Am I there yet? The views of people with learning disability on forensic community rehabilitation*. D.Clin.Psych. Thesis, University of Edinburgh.

Mcwade, B. (2014). *Recovery in an "arts for mental health" unit*. Ph.D. Thesis, Lancaster University.

Morgan, H. (2012). The social model of disability as a threshold concept: Troublesome knowledge and liminal spaces in social work education. *Social Work Education*, 31, 215–226.

Phillips, D. (2007). Embodied narratives: Control, regulation and bodily resistance in the life course of older women with learning difficulties. *European Review of History – Revue européenne d'Histoire*, 14, 503–524.

Pouncey, C. L., & Lukens, J. M. (2010). Madness versus badness: The ethical tension between the recovery movement and forensic psychiatry. *Theoretical Medicine and Bioethics*, 31, 93–105.

Reindal, S. M. (1999). Independence, dependence, interdependence: Some reflections on the subject and personal autonomy. *Disability & Society*, 14, 353–367.

Ryan, S., & Julian, G. (2015). *Actually improving care services for people with learning disabilities and challenging behaviour*. Oxford: JusticeforLB Herb Audit Office.

Shakespeare, T. (1994). Cultural representation of disabled people: Dustbins for disavowal? *Disability and Society*, 9, 283–299.

Simpson, A. I., & Penney, S. R. (2011). The recovery paradigm in forensic mental health services. *Criminal Behaviour and Mental Health*, 21, 299–306.

Thomas, C. (2006). Disability and gender: Reflections on theory and research. *Scandinavian Journal of Disability Research*, 8, 177–185.

Travers, R. (2013). *Treatment of women in forensic settings: Women and psychiatric treatment: A comprehensive text and practical guide*. London: Routledge.

Vaughn, M., & Stamp, G. H. (2003). The empowerment dilemma: The dialectic of emancipation and control in staff/client interaction at shelters for battered women. *Communication Studies*, 54, 154–168.

Williams, J. (1992). Women with learning difficulties are women too. In M. Langan & L. Day (Eds.), *Women, oppression and social work*, (pp. 149–160). London: Routledge.

Young, I. M. (2009). Five faces of oppression. In G.L. Henderson & M. Waterstone (Eds.), *Geographic Thought: A Praxis Perspective* (pp. 55–71). Oxon: Routledge.

Appendix
A Note on Methodology

This is a fuller description of my research methods and builds on the 'My ethnographic methods' section in Chapter one.

A version of this appendix has been published as:

Fish, R (2017) Researching Experiences of Learning Disabled Women on Locked Wards Using Ethnography Sage Research Methods Cases part 2 **DOI:** http://dx.doi.org/10.4135/9781526404411

I used an ethnographic method so I could see, hear and feel in context how people experience life on the locked wards and what these experiences mean to them. I did this so that I could best focus the research to be of benefit to the participants. During the ethnography, I observed the daily life of three of the flats where women were housed in a National Health Service (NHS) secure unit. The wards that I observed were designated to me by the ward manager for reasons to which I was not party. Two of the wards were classified as low secure (LSU - wards are locked but clients are able to access other areas of the unit) and one was part of the medium secure unit (MSU - wards are locked, clients must stay within the two-storey, 5.2 metre enclosure at all times). I subsequently interviewed 16 clients from those wards and 10 staff from all areas of the unit, as a follow up to the observations.

I designed my study to build on Johnson's (1998) book *Deinstitutionalising Women*, about learning disabled women living on a locked ward in Australia. For various reasons, including the way the women communicated, there are no interviews with learning disabled women documented in her book. Because all of the women in my study communicate with speech, I was able to conduct in-depth interviews and provide verbatim quotes to illustrate my arguments.

I wanted to be able to explore what people's experiences on the wards mean to them, to discover what was important to the women and staff from being in the field. As with Scior's (2003) research, I was not looking to find out what happened, but to explore the meanings given to events and how they are constructed in talk. Doing ethnography enabled me to get to know the women and also talk about the reasons as to why I was carrying out the research. It also facilitated a trusting two-way relationship. I was well aware of inequalities in the research relationship as described by feminist researchers such as Stacey (1988) - after all I was free to come and go and they were not (although they were able to refuse to participate in the research or to engage with me at all). My underlying aims were always to make recommendations that might improve the lives of women on the unit, and also to highlight *positive* aspects of daily life as described by them.

I wanted my methods to adhere to the social model of disability, where it is accepted that disability as a category is constructed socially and is a form of social oppression against disabled people (Oliver, 1990). I found that 'Inclusive research' with learning disabled people is being adopted more and more as the method of choice (e.g. Garbutt et al., 2010). Walmsley and Johnson (2003:16) suggest the following principles on which to base inclusive research:

- Research must address issues which really matter to learning disabled people, and which ultimately lead to improved lives for them;
- Research must access and represent their views and experiences;
- Learning disabled people need to be treated with respect by the research community.

Whilst planning my research, I found these principles to be crucial in enabling my accountability to the women involved. Adapting processes and environments, rather than individuals, is central to the social model of disability and I considered this adaptation to be fundamental to the practice and dissemination of my research.

Negotiating access

Prior to this project, I was employed as a part-time researcher on the unit so I knew many of the women and staff beforehand. This is not to suggest that I was a true 'insider' (Mercer, 2007) as I was not one of the direct care staff and had not visited these wards prior to the research. My lack of familiarity with daily life on the wards did, I believe, benefit the research.

In order to make sure that the research was representing the interests of the participants, one of Walmsley and Johnson's principles for inclusive research, I joined the Women's Action Group (WAG - a service user group) for 12 months prior to the research field-work, and I continued to be a member whilst the research was ongoing. The group consisted of 10 women clients and their staff, and we met every fortnight for two hours to discuss issues relevant to women living on the unit, as well as organising social and fundraising events. I described what research means and introduced the research design, analysis and dissemination with this group in order to elicit advice and opinions from the women clients and staff. This aspect was significant in the planning process; I envisaged women clients and staff having a substantial amount of input about the project through this group. However, we did not generate many suggestions, which I considered to be because of my lack of confidence in eliciting responses from the group and because of the open remit of research.

Despite my status at the time as a staff member, gaining access to the wards was still difficult and time consuming, largely due to the physical procedures of getting on and off the wards as I will describe later. I negotiated the research with management prior to commencement and in the early stages of the planning, I gained Economic and Social Research Council (ESRC) PhD studentship funding. At this point, managers were in favour of research with such an open remit being carried out. However, during the initial phases of the study, the management structure changed considerably, and further negotiations had to be done because the new managers asked for a more focussed remit. For example, they required the research to find out how women experienced certain interventions, in particular incidents of physical restraint, special observation and seclusion. This modified the focus of the study somewhat, and the interview schedule became more prescriptive than I had planned. I agreed to give feedback to the unit management and the Women's Action Group when analysis had finished. All other themes of analysis emerged from the observation and interview data.

Gaining consent for observation

My research was given ethical approval from the NHS Local Research Ethics Committee. One of the prerequisites of ethical approval was that I had to gain written consent from all the people involved, to write about any observation. This was a lengthy and difficult process, but it nevertheless enabled me to discuss the research in-depth with some people in order to gain their consent for interviews further down the line. As a feminist researcher, ethical aspects were at the forefront of my mind. I was constantly aware of issues of informed consent, and tried to explain the whole research process, including what kind of dissemination would be used, at length. The detained women who participated in the research were all labelled as having mild/moderate learning disabilities prior to admittance and were able to give consent. All participants were informed that the information that they gave would be anonymous and that their name would not be written down anywhere. I have tried to exclude any information that could identify participants, keeping in mind what measures I would want in place if I was the research participant.

My ethical adherence followed the guidance of Perry (2004). Case managers were consulted before requesting consent, and those women who were not able to give consent at the time (due to perhaps feeling extreme distress) were not part of the study; no field notes were written about situations that they were involved in. Verbal checks were performed with clients to make sure they had understood the process of the research.

At the observation stage, I felt that observing more than one ward would help to ensure anonymity when disseminating the research internally. If any woman became very distressed or disturbed during that time, the managers agreed to inform me. Most women were able to consent, but on the MSU there were two women who were newly admitted and were being looked after away from the others and it was quite obvious to me not to approach them.

A meeting with staff and clients was arranged before the participant observation began to assure them that all field notes and other records would be anonymised.

All clients and staff on the ward were given an information sheet telling them about the objectives of the observation. Separate consent forms were completed for staff and clients, and for participation in the observation and interviews. The consent form assured participants that all their data would be kept confidential, unless they divulged that they or someone else were in danger of/or being harmed. Any participant who disclosed at this point that they had been subject to abuse was referred for counselling if the issue had not been already acknowledged and addressed. Any client or staff member who did not agree to be observed was not written about in the field notes and was informed about this (there was only one staff member who declined). I spent time on the wards and at day services with staff and clients, making sure that observations were unobtrusive and unthreatening and fieldnotes were not written in visibility of any clients or staff. Fieldnotes were typed up afterwards, anonymised on transcription, and password protected.

Carrying out the interviews

My observations produced many fieldnotes, which I arranged into themes. I developed interview questions/themes as a result of this stage of the data collection and subsequently I carried out in-depth interviews. I interviewed both staff and service users, and all interviewees had a great deal of scope for determining the direction and topics of the interview, for instance many of the questions were open ended and general, such as, 'How do you feel about living here?' and 'How do you think services for women could be improved?' All participants in the observation phase of the research were invited to be interviewed, and although one member of staff and two clients declined, ten staff and sixteen clients agreed to be involved. All were white British and between the ages of 18 and 60 (as are most staff and clients at the Unit).

At the interview stage, clients who had been involved in the observation were approached on the ward and given the information sheet which was read together with them. A consent form was used, with relevant checks for understanding. For example, the consent form specified that the participant could withdraw from the study at any time without recrimination, and that this would not affect their treatment or care in any way, and they would not have to give a reason for withdrawing. This was read out to the participant and then if I was uncertain that it had been understood, I asked a question to check understanding, for example – 'What will happen if you want to drop out of the study?' All clients had information presented verbally in an accessible manner, and were also given an information form to take away which was presented in pictorial and easy-read information to aid understanding. The full research process was explained to participants in order that they knew exactly what would happen to their information after the interviews.

The interview information forms specified that all information given would be audio recorded and stored on a computer, where it would be anonymised on transcription and any potentially identifying information would not be typed. Also included on the consent form was the condition that if the participant disclosed that they or others were being harmed in any way, or if they were likely to harm themselves or others, this would be passed on to their case manager in a confidential and sensitive manner. Only the research supervisors and I had access to the transcripts, and this information was included on the information sheet.

I was constantly aware that informed consent is an ongoing process and must be regularly discussed and checked. If the participant agreed to be involved in further interviews, at the beginning of each interview, their willingness to remain involved was checked verbally.

Interviews were based around just five questions:

- How do clients and staff experience day-to-day life on the wards?
- What do women clients value about the service?
- How do women feel they are progressing through the service?
- How do women clients and staff experience and perceive the staff/client relationship in this environment?
- How do staff and clients experience physical intervention, seclusion and enhanced observation?

The recommendations from Unit C's management that obliged me to explore the subjects of seclusion, special observations and physical intervention meant I was compelled to introduce these subjects even if participants did not. However, I soon found that the interviews flowed better if I asked one or two questions and then prompted the participants for further information, so that they were introducing the themes of the interview themselves. I found that many of the participants did this, and I would just probe further into each theme that I wanted to look at. For example, when a participant started to speak about seclusion or physical restraint, I would probe this, saying something like, 'So, you mentioned being put into seclusion, how did that feel?'

This relates again to Walmsley and Johnson's principles for inclusive research, the participants had significant influence over what we talked about and how much they said about it, and sometimes would choose not to answer a question. I was constantly aware of my ethical responsibility with regard to both the observation and the interviews. I considered doing ethical research to be more important than collecting data, as Booth and Booth (2005) also recommend in their work.

I found the interviews with clients to be very successful, with a few clients commenting how much they enjoyed being interviewed and how it was good to get things off their chest. They had much to say about the service and were very open and honest. I think this is due to the rapport I built up with clients during the WAG and the observations in the flats, which I acknowledge has been to the cost of any rapport with staff. Some writers (e.g. Goffman, 1961) agree that a researcher has to be partisan to one group or another within the research field, and I demonstrated more interest in engaging with the clients than the staff. Time spent with the staff would have been at the expense of spending time with the clients; my time on the flats was always limited. Nonetheless, I did observe many interactions between staff and clients and got to know a lot more about what the staff do on the wards, as well as conduct interviews with them. I do hope, therefore, that this work will be to the benefit of both groups.

Many of the things I was told as a researcher were difficult to hear, and I felt privileged to be in the trusted situation that allowed this, but also conscious that I was using this trust as a way to get a PhD and advance my own career. Disengaging myself from these relationships that had been built up was difficult (Rogers, 2003) but was made easier by my leaving to go on maternity leave. I subsequently provided staff and client reports and presentations about the research for the organisation.

Other ethical issues

It was decided that external dissemination and publications would not include the name of the service or any of the participants. Ethical researchers must carefully consider the potential benefits of their research and for whom these benefits arise (Griffin et al., 2004), and although this research may not in the future necessarily have a *directly* positive impact on the participants, I consider it important to disseminate the results and recommendations widely and in an accessible way to all participants and policymakers.

Ethical review involved completing an extensive online form, attaching information sheets and consent forms for each stage of the research and for each group (staff and clients). As mentioned earlier, I attended an NHS Research Ethics Committee to introduce the research and answer questions. The members of the ethics committee were very concerned about the ethnography, asking many questions about what I was going to be doing during my time on the wards and what would happen if I witnessed instances of inappropriate care. They recommended numerous changes to the information and consent forms and I had to amend these forms twice before I was granted ethical approval. I did feel that the research needed to be articulated in a certain way to get through ethics and local approval procedures, for example I was often asked what my hypothesis was, and the ethics forms asked for specific research questions and outcomes from the research. The whole process from completion of the form to ethical approval took six months.

When the research project had been agreed and ethical approval obtained, I arranged to visit each of the two wards during one day per week at different times to observe daily life there. I found this 'getting to know each other' period to be invaluable in gaining both clients' and staff's trust and subsequently, meaningful interviews, however I was constantly wary of the ethical aspects and power imbalances in the research relationship (Stacey, 1988). I also found that spending time with people allowed me to explain the research project in much more detail to participants who might not easily understand the complexities of research.

Building of friendships was difficult to avoid and there were a few instances where one of the clients 'took me under her wing' and I did spend more time with some of the women rather than others. I was always careful not to exploit the relationships I had built up, and kept in mind that my main research objective was to make recommendations which could improve the lives of women clients and staff on the wards.

The hardest part of the observation was gaining access physically to the wards. Each time I went to the low secure wards (LSU), I had to ring a bell to have the door clicked open remotely, and then someone had to come and unlock the internal doors with a key to let me in. I often had to explain about the research to a different person on the desk and was usually asked who I wanted to see. On the medium secure unit, I had to wait to enter a 'bubble': a space contained by two locked doors which cannot both be unlocked together. Then I had to give a key card with my identification on it through a hatch which looks like a bank till. In return, I got a belt with a pouch and a bunch of keys on a nylon webbing strap with an electronic fob to unlock certain doors and a personal alarm. After organising these items onto the belt and pouch, I was let through into the MSU. Having keys allowed me to access different areas and take clients to a range of rooms, including day services.

I spent over 120 hours observing the life on the wards at different times of the day, over a period of nine months. My time on the wards involved much sitting and talking; many of the women said they were happy to have someone to talk to who did not have the duties of other staff. I purposefully did not spend too much time talking with staff on the wards, so that the women would not consider me to have a supervisory role. I do believe that my presence did influence what happened on the wards, for example there was very little conflict between the women whilst I was there despite this being a significant theme in the interviews. Although there may have been many reasons for this, I believe that this detail demonstrates that the process of observation stimulated important themes to emerge during interviews. The fact that conflict was reduced during my time on the wards also seemingly reflects my status as a partial 'outsider', something which ensured that very little was taken for granted as the field was all new to me. Hopefully this enabled the data to be rich and accessible to the reader.

During the interview stage, I found that women who knew me through the observational period and through my membership of the WAG group were much more likely to talk in-depth than women with whom I had little contact. One woman, for example, agreed to be interviewed but started to feel anxious and stopped the interview after about 8 minutes. This woman was somebody I hadn't had much contact with and I was concerned about how the interview progressed. Most of the clients were very happy to talk in an interview, especially during times of little activity such as early evening or just before the evening meal. Staff are needed at all times, however, so staff in both areas were difficult to pin down to be interviewed. There was often too few staff to allow one to leave the ward, or go to a separate room, and asking staff to be interviewed during their hard-earned break or after a 13-hour shift seemed excessive. Observations carried on during the interview phase and the whole of my fieldwork lasted 11 months altogether.

Spending time on the wards was enjoyable, but also distressing, intense and sometimes daunting. I had some fun with the clients and staff, but seeing clients and staff feeling angry, spending time with weeping clients who had just self-harmed, and listening to some stories from people's pasts was extremely distressing. I was always aware of Stacey's (1988) comments about people's lives merely translating into research data, and when women told me about the bad times in their lives I asked them if I could include it in the research. Usually the answer was 'yes, as long as you take my name out.' Further, I was worried about how I was going to represent the women (staff and clients) in the unit. I didn't want to 'other' the women clients myself by reinforcing gender and disability norms, or represent the staff as aloof or cold-hearted. Representation of people is a big responsibility and one I didn't take lightly, but I do acknowledge that my subjectivity and past experiences will affect my interpretations and how I write about people. Certain material was left out of the data because of my commitment to ethical research and writing.

Analysis

The fieldnotes and interview transcripts were all uploaded to a qualitative software package, NVIVO to aid with the management of such large amounts of data. I borrowed my analysis method from the phenomenological research tradition (Hycner, 1985) and followed the steps suggested by Hycner in order that the analysis was inductive, arising from the data. I read through the transcriptions many times to make myself aware of emerging themes, making sure that I was not overlooking any themes due to my preconceptions. Each item of text in NVIVO is given a label (the title of the theme), and it is possible to run a query to draw out all text relating to that label. At first, there were a large number of labels, but then it became possible to group them under 'umbrella' terms, for example, the themes 'being away from family' and 'family visits' could be grouped under the term 'family relationships'. Being able to read all the information in a theme was very useful, as it allowed me to have an overview of what people were saying about the topic and develop conceptual questions from this data.

During the analysis stage, Hycner recommends a process called 'bracketing', which involves putting your ideas to one side by recognising how your life experiences and preconceptions might affect interpretation. I consider this to be an impossible endeavour; despite attempting to be as faithful to the participants' experiences as possible, I acknowledge that the data will always be interpreted through my eyes. For example, my fieldnotes describe what I noticed in my time on the wards, and my opinions of these situations, and what I noticed and judged to be important will be contingent on my knowledge and life experiences. Furthermore, I have chosen which themes to include in the book, which themes are most important to report, and although I have tried to introduce as many as possible, I acknowledge that all interpretations are related to me in some way.

Conclusion

A Disability Studies approach might argue that research should focus entirely on disabled people themselves, rather than carers, support workers or medical professionals. I suggest in contrast that unless research examines the relationships and differing perspectives in institutions like the one in which the women in my study are forced to live, we cannot adequately understand the difficulties and challenges some disabled people face on a daily basis.

Learning disabled people are rarely asked about their opinions of residential services, and the fact that these women are incarcerated means that they may be even less likely to feel able to express their views about where they live and how they are treated. Although clients were mostly welcoming and happy to have me around, my research began during a well-publicised police inquiry into the abuse of learning disabled people in a private residential service (Winterbourne View). For this reason, I am aware that some staff were suspicious of my presence on the ward and may have felt that I was spying on them. My experience of trying to involve people in the progress of the research by joining the women's group (WAG) was also not very successful as I have mentioned. The women listened when I talked about the research, but they understandably found it difficult to respond to questions about the direction of research. Although this attempt at getting people involved was not particularly effective, I felt that using ethnography to understand the women's everyday lives was enough to ensure that their opinions and experiences were represented. Nevertheless, joining the WAG was useful in getting to know potential research participants, and updating them on the research as it went on.

I think that that my choice of method fulfilled the principles of *inclusive* research, despite not achieving client involvement throughout in terms of design and analysis. I hope the themes I address will translate into policy, benefitting both staff and clients in some way. I remain in favour of *emancipatory* research, but I argue that for any projects on the unit to be classed as emancipatory, they would be very time consuming and would require a group of people to meet regularly to focus on planning the research and the provision of training in research skills to clients. Clients would have to learn much more about what research involves, which was not appropriate within the time and ethical constraints of the PhD study on which this book is based. I feel that inclusive research was sufficient in terms of being faithful to the stories of the detained women.

Although the planning and early stages of the research were time consuming and difficult, and despite the obstacles I have described, I maintain that my method was the most appropriate and effective as time allowed: women clients and staff had control over the research focus and I was able to observe what was important to them, the meaning they gave to everyday experiences in the Unit. I was able to use a Disability Studies approach, in that I could adapt my questions to my participants' communication style and ability. I also adhered to feminist values by acknowledging all my participants as equals and not privileging any voice over another. I would recommend this methodology to all researchers working in these fields.

Bibliography

Booth, T. & Booth, W. 2005. Parents with learning difficulties in the child protection system. *Journal of Intellectual Disabilities,* 9, 109.

Garbutt, R., Tattersall, J., Dunn, J. & Boycott-Garnett, R. 2010. Accessible article: involving people with learning disabilities in research. *British Journal of Learning Disabilities,* 38, 21–34.

Griffin, T., Balandin, S., Emerson, E., Hatton, C., Thompson, T. & Parmenter, T. 2004. Ethical research involving people with intellectual disabilities. *The international handbook of applied research in intellectual disabilities,* 61–82.

Hycner, R. H. 1985. Some guidelines for the phenomenological analysis of interview data. *Human studies,* 8, 279–303.

Johnson, K. 1998. *Deinstitutionalising women: an ethnographic study of institutional closure,* Cambridge Univ Pr.

Mercer, J. 2007. The challenges of insider research in educational institutions: Wielding a double-edged sword and resolving delicate dilemmas. *Oxford Review of Education,* 33, 1–17.

Oliver, M. 1990. The individual and social models of disability. *Royal College of Physicians.* London.

Perry, J. 2004. Interviewing people with intellectual disabilities. *In:* EMERSON, E., HATTON, C., THOMPSON, J. & PARMENTER, T. (eds.) *The international handbook of applied research in intellectual disabilities.* Chichester: Wiley.

Rogers, C. 2003. The mother/researcher in blurred boundaries of a reflexive research process. *Auto/Biography,* 11, 47–54.

Scior, K. 2003. Using discourse analysis to study the experiences of women with learning disabilities. *Disability & Society,* 18, 779–795.

Stacey, J. 1988. Can there be a feminist ethnography? *Women's Studies International Forum,* 11, 21–27.

Walmsley, J. & Johnson, K. 2003. *Inclusive research with people with learning disabilities: past, present, and futures,* London, Jessica Kingsley.

Index

For Product Safety Concerns and Information please contact our
EU representative GPSR@taylorandfrancis.com Taylor & Francis
Verlag GmbH, Kaufingerstraße 24, 80331 München, Germany